Functions
Of A
Manager
In Occupational Therapy

Revised Edition

Functions
Of A
Manager
In Occupational Therapy

Revised Edition

Edited by

Karen Jacobs, EdD, OTR/L, FAOTA
Martha K. Logigian, MS, OTR/L

ABZ-0071

Managing Editor: Amy E. Drummond
Cover Design: Linda Baker
Publisher: John Bond

Printed in the United States of America

ISBN 1-55642-216-4

Published by: SLACK Incorporated
                6900 Grove Road
                Thorofare, NJ 08086-9447

Last digit is print number: 10 9 8 7 6 5 4 3 2 1

Dedication

To Future Occupational Therapy Managers

Contents

Acknowledgments

Appreciation is due everyone who assisted in the preparation of this textbook. Our publisher, SLACK Incorporated, has our appreciation for its assistance. Specifically, we would like to thank Harry Benson, who supported the concept of this book and helped make it a reality, and Amy Drummond and Debra Clarke, who offered editorial assistance. Finally, our thanks are extended to our families for their love and support. K.J. & M.L.

Preface to Revised Edition

Since 1989, much has changed in the health care arena. The climate in the United States is changing and we all await the impact of President Clinton's health care reform. It has become crucial for occupational therapists to have a good understanding of the functions of a manager during these times. This revised edition of Functions of a Manager contains ten chapters, all of which have been rewritten or updated to reflect our health care climate. In addition, we have added a chapter on developing new programs.

Preface to First Edition

The theme of this textbook for undergraduate occupational therapy students is the functions of a manager, including those of a planner, director, organizer, budgeter, supervisor, and leader. Being a manager is a role that many occupational therapists assume during the courses of their careers. By providing information on the functions of a manager during the years of formal education, we hope to introduce and foster the enjoyment and importance of this role. This book is designed to address ten functions of a manager organized into macro and micro-management environments. The macro-environment includes Chapter 1: Managing Human Resources; Chapter 2: Management Information Systems; Chapter 3: Marketing Occupational Therapy Services; Chapter 4: Ethical Issues in Occupational Therapy; and Chapter 5: Supervision. The micro-environment includes Chapter 6: Cost Management; Chapter 7: Documentation in Health Care; Chapter 8: Designing Fieldwork Programs; Chapter 9: Quality Management in Occupational Therapy and Chapter 10: Developing a New Occupational Therapy Program. Use of this textbook has been facilitated by the provision of two case studies and multiple choice questions at the end of each chapter.

Contributing Authors

Gail M. Bloom, MA, OTR/L, Executive Director, The Samaritans of the Merrimack Valley Methuen, MA Instructor, Mt. Ida College, Newton, MA

Ellen S. Cohn, EdM, OTR/L, FAOTA, Academic Fieldwork Coordinator, Tufts University, Boston School of Occupational Therapy, Medford, MA

Jan Johnston Gannon, MBA, OTR/L, President of Board of Directors, Shelburne Children's Center, Shelburne, VT

Bette Hoffman Harel, MS, OTR/L, Industrial Consultant, Workwright, Inc., Needham, MA

Karen Jacobs, EdD, OTR/L, FAOTA, Clinical Assistant Professor, Boston University Department of Occupational Therapy, Boston, MA

Martha K. Logigian, MS, OTR/L, Director of Rehabilitation Services, Brigham and Women's Hospital, Boston, MA

Janice F. Pagonis, MS, OTR/L, Therapist, Oakland Rehabilitation Associates, Pittsburgh, PA

Rita A. Parisi, OTR/L, Administrative Director, Center for Rehabilitation, Berkshire Medical Center, Berkshire, MA

Laurel Cargill Radley, MS, OTR, Occupational Therapist, Fairfield, ME

Mary Jane Youngstrom, MS, OTR/L, Assistant Professor, Kansas City University Department of Occupational Therapy, Kansas City, KS

CHAPTER 1

Managing Human Resources

Rita A. Parisi, OTR/L

Introduction

The primary objective of this chapter is to discuss the role of a supervisor in managing human resources, specifically recruitment and retention of employees. To manage that process effectively it is necessary to integrate and implement many management concepts. Important concepts include:

- Marketing management
- Managing organization and individual behavior
- Understanding what motivates employees
- Developing effective communication
- Understanding individual and group dynamics
- Developing leadership skills

Recruiting and retaining health care professionals has become increasingly difficult during the past 10 years. It will be one of the most difficult issues that department managers will have to face in the 1990s. In the 1970s much of the literature that analyzed and predicted career trends projected tremendous growth in the need for therapy providers. Unfortunately, from the perspective of a department manager, the number of clinicians does not meet the need for therapy services, creating a supply and demand problem. To grasp a full understanding of the issue, the following brief historical information is provided. A literature review revealed the following major reasons for increased demand of therapy services.

1. Growth of rehabilitation because of increased public awareness and push for increased independence of handicapped/disabled individuals.
2. Trend of using highly trained nonphysician professionals to provide services previously provided by physicians.
3. Federal and state regulations that demand therapy services for target populations. For example, children between the ages of 3 and 21 with identified needs.
4. Increased Medicare and Medicaid coverage for occupational therapy services provided in outpatient and home health settings.
5. Increased emphasis on health care promotion and prevention therapy creating new employment markets that require occupational therapy services. For example, walk-in clinics and sports medicine clinics.
6. The aging of America, which creates an increased number of elderly who are major users of therapy services.

Recruitment

Health care business trends usually are behind other business industry trends. Recruitment methods utilized in health care are not exceptions to that rule. Therefore, a health care manager can learn a great deal by exploring recruitment methods utilized by other industries. Managers can relate those methods to their organizations.

Recruitment can be approached from a marketing perspective. Marketing is simply defined as understanding the consumer's needs so that the product is seen as having value to the consumer: in marketing it is important to clearly define the product, price, and sales/promotion plan to the consumer. The same ideas can be generalized to recruitment. The applicant is the consumer, the product is the facility and/or organization, the price is the salary and benefit package, and the sales/promotion plan is a method utilized to attract applicants. Therefore, from a marketing perspective, it is important to do the following:

1. Identify the applicant's or consumer's potential needs. For example, many clinicians are women who have young children. Flexible hours and child care might be important to their needs. Other needs might be laddering opportunities, education, and so on.
2. Define the product in terms of the facility/organization's strengths and unique characteristics.
3. Define the price or salary and benefit package. If the applicant is considering employment at the facility, the salary and benefits need to be competitive and of value to the consumer or applicant. This idea is similar to the consumer who needs to feel a product is worth the price for which it is selling.
4. Develop a sales/promotion plan that is needed to attract applicants and sell them on employment.

Health care recruiters and recruitment companies are showing tremendous growth. Ten years ago less than 5% of therapy providers were introduced to their jobs via recruiters. That figure has grown significantly over the past ten years. In fact, many health care organizations have hired recruiters. The recruitment process has become very costly and frustrating to many organizations.

Following are six basic steps in the recruitment process:

- Define the job and qualifications
- Attract applicants
- Set up an interview
- Check references
- Offer the job
- Follow up the worker's progress

Job Definition

The job definition is an important step that requires more attention than it is usually given. It is of vital importance to match the applicant with the job. It is impossible to do that without a clear understanding of the job the applicant is being recruited for. As we all know, the role of the occupational therapist varies in each setting. Therefore it is important to have a job description for the position that is being recruited.

A job description should contain the following elements:

- Title of job
- Organizational relationship—include in this section whom the individual reports to and the kind and degree of supervision received. Also include who this individual coordinates with and supervises
- Summary of primary functions
- Work performed—describe specific duties indicating the importance of each
- Job requirements—include specific skills and education required to perform the job
- Significant environmental risks—includes hazards of the position, e.g., back injuries from lifting, exposure to diseases

After a job description is completed it is important to translate the duties in the general job description into individual specifications. A job description does not always tell what to look for in a candidate. Individualized specifications might include personality characteristics, past experience and accomplishments.[1,4,10]

Methods to Attract Applicants

Look at methods utilized to attract applicants from short- and long-run perspectives. It is very important to present a positive image and keep your organization's name in front of prospective candidates.

Successful short-run methods in attracting applicants include the following:

- Sponsor open house events that invite clinicians to the facility
- Place an eye-catching ad in recruitment journals and/or newspapers
- Offer incentive bonuses to employees who recruit their friends and classmates to work at the facility
- Attend recruitment fairs sponsored by recruitment forums
- Attend professional conferences for the purpose of recruiting, not education
- Send recruitment letters to clinicians' homes
- Send out informational papers to local clinicians
- Encourage staff to write articles on clinical programs offered in the facility to be placed in recruitment newspapers

Methods utilized to keep attracting applicants in the long run do not usually yield immediate rewards. Because it is hard to show immediate benefits of these efforts, many shortsighted organizations might not value the time invested. Our experience confirms that the time spent in these methods is just as valuable as the time invested in short-run methods. Activities used to attract applicants in the long run are as follows:

- Provide lectures to colleges and universities that have occupational therapy programs
- Participate in high school career days to promote the profession and make direct contact with students
- Encourage staff to present papers at national and local education forums
- Train occupational therapy students at the facility
- Build networking channels within the profession by participating in state organization and special interest groups
- Send out educational mailing on a regular basis

Interviews

Once there are applicants, the interview process begins. It is important to prepare for the interview. The interview style can be directive and formal or nondirective and informal. The manager needs to decide which style is most comfortable and which will obtain the information the manager needs. This is the time to set mutual expectations. Active listening skills are a must for interviewing. The objectives of an interview are to determine the following:

- Is the applicant a match for your organization and job description?
- Do the applicant's technical skills match the organization's needs?
- What are the applicant's career goals?
- Does the applicant's working style match the environment?
- Is the applicant interested in working at the facility?

The shortage of clinicians has created a situation where the applicants are usually interviewing at several facilities at the same time. The manager should consider giving the applicant written information to take when leaving. It is important for the manager to highlight the strengths and unique characteristics of the organization. Meeting the key individuals other than the department manager might be useful and allows the applicant to gain a better perspective about the organization. It also gives the manager opportunities to solicit opinions from others regarding the applicant's potential.[2,8,9]

Reference Check

It is important to check references on applicants to whom you are planning to offer a job. The increasing shortage of clinicians and desire to fill vacancies might influence a department manager to skip this step. This is not a good idea because the information obtained on a reference check assists the manager in making an informed decision. It is not always possible to determine if an applicant is a good match for your job based on an interview. It is more costly to hire an individual who does not match the job and organization's goals.

Reference checks can be performed on the telephone or by mail. Telephone references are faster than mail references. The telephone also can allow more flexibility than a written reference. A written reference usually requires less time from the manager to obtain information.

Job Offer

The department manager usually makes the job offer to the potential employee. The job offer should include terms of employment, salary, and an agreement on starting date.

Follow Up

Once a verbal agreement has been reached between the potential new employee and department manager, write a letter to the new employee. The letter should contain a welcome to the organization, salary, starting date, work hours, documents necessary for first day of work, and any other information that would be helpful to a new employee. For example, the dress code, parking and public transit, and types of food available on-site to the employee.

If more than one month passes between the job offer and starting date, a phone call might be worthwhile. Many individuals have ambivalent feelings when leaving one employer and going to another. Therefore, a phone call confirming the job offer might reassure the new employee.

Retention

It is important to be successful at recruitment, but success at retention is more important. The way the clinician is assimilated into the organization plays a major role in retention of that employee. The employee's early experiences in the organization can significantly affect job satisfaction, employee attitude, productivity, and turnover.

The psychological contract—setting of expectations and matching of the individual's and organization's goals—begins during the interview process.[11] Once a new employee is scheduled to begin working, each manager struggles with setting up priorities about how much work time versus training time is expected. The training time can vary depending on the work experience the new employee has. Training time might be minimal if the department has been short staffed and there is a lot of work waiting for the new employee.

The orientation process has both formal and informal components. The formal process attempts to assimilate the new employee into the organization and give the employee a common base of reference and resources. It sends a message to new employees that their understanding of each department and the facility as a whole is important. The informal welcoming process is just as important for the individual to learn the informal channels in the organization.

The following are recommendations to successfully recruit and retain employees in the organization:

1. **Match**—Managers should match the employee's strengths with the first assignment, have written material available for reference, and balance new employee's work schedule between initiating the job and the orientation process.

2. **Training**—Each manager should internally review the priorities of the balance of orientation and training process versus job productivity expectations. An appropriate amount of time spent training an employee pays off in less time and higher job performance in the long run. The employee that has just been hired is on your payroll because you hired him or her, and because you want that employee to be a productive, efficient member of your unit. You want to develop the new employee into someone who measures up to your standards of performance.

The following are some thoughts to keep in mind about what individuals want their jobs to be:

- Most clinicians want to do well on their job and desire to excel in the new employment
- Clinicians want to believe their jobs are important. It is necessary to continue to convince the clinicians at the start that you are counting on them and will help them attain the skills necessary to perform their jobs well[1,9]
- Clinicians like to perform a job that shows results. It is important to help clinicians see the value of their contribution to the organization. They need to understand that they are not just filling a void[4]
- Most clinicians like to work for a manager who sets high standards that are challenging but attainable
- A training program should establish an environment that will encourage the new clinician to do the best in learning the job, set standards of performance and give the clinician an opportunity to demonstrate abilities. As managers you should check often to show you are interested in the clinician's progress

3. Job Expectations—Clear job expectations need to be established. Specific criteria performance expectations need to be clear to clinicians. Criteria based performance systems might help establish clear expectations.

4. Orientation—Each clinician should participate in a formal orientation process. A manager understands that effective orientation takes planning. The following checklist might be helpful to plan an effective orientation program:

- Establish the right environment
- Explain the orientation and training program
- Make appropriate introductions and take the clinician on a tour of the department
- Tell the clinician how the job is integrated into the organization as a whole
- Review administrative rules and regulations
- Follow up regularly, especially the first week
- Do not keep unsatisfactory clinicians in the department. If you are convinced the new clinician is not able to achieve the minimum performance expectations, do not put off the inevitable

5. Informal Welcoming Process—Structuring of the informal welcoming process might help managers improve their skills in this area. We each get caught in the hectic pace of daily operations and might not take the time to converse with the new employees. The assignment of a senior worker in a "buddy system" also can help the new employee feel welcomed.

6. Motivation—Managers should examine what motivates their employees. There are many theories as to what motivates employees. Most theorists agree that understanding employee motivation involves a variety of individual and organizational factors. The organizational factors include the job, pay, recognition, and job security. The individual factors include needs, abilities, goals, and attitude. Managers need to match rewards to the factors that motivate their employees. Rewards can be financial, promotions, and/or recognition.[1,11]

7. Supervision—Check on the clinician's performance via regular supervision meetings to allow for regular feedback for performance appraisal. Taking the time to work with new employees sends the message to clinicians that the quality of their performance is important. Ensure the performance appraisal process is more than a once a year event. Management by an objective performance review system allows for more staff participation than traditional performance review systems.[4,5]

Career development is a continuous process. A supervisor can be instrumental in assisting an employee to achieve career goals. Career development is a selection and growth process that takes place between individuals and their employers. It should be a process of matching individual and organizational needs over time.[3] It takes conscious effort on the part of employee and supervisor to develop the employee's skills and match them with organizational needs. This match can only occur when the employee and the organization know each other's needs and expectations. Individuals go through stages in developing their careers: growth, exploration, establishment, maintenance, and decline.[11] Open communication and employees establishing their own goals during a performance appraisal process will help in matching and knowing each other's career goals if the supervisor understands what career stage the employee is in.

8. Benefits—It is important to develop a benefit package that meets the needs of employees. A flexible benefit package allows the opportunity to meet a variety of needs. Major benefits to consider are health, dental, education, childcare, and time off.[7]

Conclusion

In summary, recruitment and retention have become major and important job responsibilities for department managers. A manager who effectively manages these processes needs to understand how to manage human resources—especially how to integrate the concepts of marketing, employee motivation, effective communication, and how to manage organization and individual behavior.

Questions

1. The psychological contract formed between an employer and an employee begins:
   a. First day of work
   b. At the time of the first performance review
   c. During the interview process
   d. At the end of the probationary period

2. A job description contains which of the following categories:
   a. Personality characteristics necessary to perform job
   b. Organizational chart
   c. Dress code
   d. Organizational relationships to job

3. A definition of marketing is:
   a. Understanding the consumer's needs so the potential products have value to the consumer
   b. Selling products to the consumer
   c. Determining the price of a product
   d. Public relations

4. Career stages individuals go through include the following (circle all of the appropriate answers):
   a. Training
   b. Establishment
   c. Decline
   d. Growth

5. Professional networking for the department manager is important for:
   a. Visibility
   b. Recruitment
   c. Retention
   d. Getting ahead

6. High turnover might be a result of:
   a. Training
   b. Matching of rewards to what factors motivate employees
   c. Formal orientation
   d. Mismatching of employee and employer expectations

7. Which of the following are parts of the recruitment process:
   a. Job definition
   b. Performance appraisal
   c. Orientation
   d. Welcome process

8. Employee career development can be enhanced via:
   a. Employer benefit packages that meet employee's needs
   b. Supervisor and employee working together to develop employee's skills to match them with organization's needs
   c. Clearly defining the job
   d. Informal orientation process

9. Employee's early experiences in the organization can affect (circle all of the appropriate answers):
   a. Career growth patterns of employee
   b. The psychological contract established between the employee and employer
   c. Employee productivity
   d. Turnover

10. Identification of potential applicant's needs to attract applicants and the employer's attempts to meet those needs is a_____ approach to recruitment.
    a. Shortsighted
    b. Production
    c. Marketing
    d. Business

Answers
1. c
2. d
3. a
4. a, c, d
5. b
6. d
7. a
8. b
9. b, c, d
10. c

Case Study 1

Betty Block has been an occupational therapist for five years. Her current job is a senior staff position in a small acute care hospital. She provides both inpatient and outpatient services. Betty is a very committed and loyal employee. The hospital she works for administratively organized several departments including occupational therapy. The occupational therapy director's position was vacant because of the resignation of the director four months previously. Betty had consciously decided not to pursue the director's position. Her reasons were her disinterest in supervising others and an interest in emphasizing further development of her clinical skills. In the reorganization, the occupational therapy director's position was eliminated. The occupational therapy staff now reports to Betty, who reports to the director of physical therapy. She is expected to provide clinical supervision to four OTRs as well as carry three-fourths of a caseload. Betty's job satisfaction has significantly decreased. The physical therapy director's management style is very different than the previous director's style. Betty has only had a few supervising meetings with the new boss. Betty assumes her boss is aware of the dissatisfaction. What should Betty do?

Betty experienced high job satisfaction until six months ago. Her job expectations changed with very little communication between her and her boss. Betty's job expectations no longer meet her employer's. The psychological contract between Betty and her employer has been broken. Her new boss has not established a new contract. Betty is an experienced clinician. She is responsible for communicating her needs to her boss. If Betty is unable to renegotiate her psychological contract she needs to decide if she wants to make a job change. Change in an organization is inevitable unless the organization operates in a vacuum. As change occurs it is important to renegotiate expectations between the employer and employee. Successful reintegration can take place if the parties involved communicate well. If Betty decides to pursue employment elsewhere, she needs to prepare for interviewing.

Case Study 2

The OT department at JFF Hospital experienced 50% turnover and an inability to recruit clinicians. The OT director was extremely frustrated and unsure what actions she should take to reduce turnover and successfully recruit. The director consulted with the hospital's resource department.

The following suggestions were made:

- Identify the reason(s) for high turnover rate. A simple way to obtain that information is to ask the clinicians who left why they did
- Develop a retention plan utilizing information obtained from the former employees
- Develop a recruitment plan that includes short- and long-term recruitment ideas

The information received from former employees that the OT director felt she could control revealed:

- Desire to change work schedule so other career opportunities can be pursued
- Dissatisfaction because of lack of career opportunities and lack of recognition
- Staff felt administration had unrealistic workload expectations of them.

Based on that information the director worked with her supervisory staff to better meet the staff's needs. They developed a plan to provide more professional growth opportunities for staff and increased recognition. The management group worked with the staff on renegotiation of workload expectations. The negotiation process helped to increase the staff's understanding of the expectations. A plan to implement a criteria based management by objective performance appraisal system developed. That system would assist staff to take more control of their work schedule. It also provided more direction to the supervisors to help staff achieve their career goals. A plan also was developed to allow more flexible work hours.

A short-run and long-run assessment plan was developed and implemented. The plan included placing an eye-catching ad in a recruitment paper that identified strengths and unique characteristics. Members of the department attended conferences with the purpose of recruiting, not just education. Development of a student program met both retention and recruitment needs of the department.

The director wrote the job descriptions and expectations for the vacant jobs to ensure setting appropriate job expectations with any potential applicants during the interview process.

The director set time frames to assess her success and/or lack of success with her new recruitment and retention plans.

References

1. Ploynick M, Rubin I, & Fry R. *Managing Human Resources in Healthcare Organizations*: Reston Publishing Co. Reston, Virginia, 1978.
2. Porter M. *Competitive Strategy—Techniques for Analyzing Industries and Competitors*: MacMillan Publisher. New York, New York, 1980.
3. Truskie S. Manager's Journal: New York, NY: *Wall Street Journal*, 1981.
4. Middlebrook B & Rachel F. Performance Appraisals: Much More Than Once a Year Task: *Supervisory Management*, September 1982.
5. Wiatrowski M & Palkon F. Performance Appraisal System in Healthcare Administration: *Healthcare Manage Review* 12(1), 71-80, 1987.
6. Shell B & Kieshauer M. Managing for Performance. AJOT 41(5), May 1987.
7. Wyrick J & Stern E. Recruitment of OT Students: A National Survey. AJOT 41(3), March 1987.
8. Koen C. The Pre-Employment Inquiry Guide. Costa Mesa, CA: *Personnel Journal*, October 1980.
9. Peters T & Waterman Jr. R. *In Search of Excellence*. New York, NY. Harper & Row Publishers, 1982.
10. Newman W, Warren E & McGill A. *The Process of Management*. Englewood Cliffs, NJ: Prentice Hall, 1987.
11. Chung K & Megginson L. *Organizational Behavior*. New York, NY: Harper & Row Publishers, 1981.
12. Kotler P. *Marketing Management*. Englewood Cliffs, NJ: Prentice-Hall, Inc., 1984.

CHAPTER 2

Management Information Systems

Jan Johnston Gannon, MBA, OTR/L

Introduction

Man lives in a very complex environment that can be "viewed as a dynamic, ongoing, ever-changing interaction of conditions and observations that result in subsequent responses."[4] The conditions are the events and activities that occur based on the composition of the environment. To interpret these conditions, observations are made and recorded by a sensory device, human or machine. The subsequent response is based upon an evaluation and analysis of the observed conditions. Man constantly uses sensory information from the environment to formulate an appropriate response.[4]

The number of conditions man must observe, resulting in a multitude of alternative actions, is often so extensive that it is beyond one's capacity to process such information. Even if it is within man's realm to work on such information, sacrifices are made in timeliness, quality, and accuracy of the resulting decision. Therefore, to process the vast quantity of information available, information systems must be developed to help retain all necessary information.

What is an Information System?

Before discussing the types of information systems available, it is crucial to define exactly what information is. To define information, one must first understand the difference between data, as the raw material, and information, as the end product. Data can be defined as "any experience, proceeding an occurrence that is the result of direct observation or perception by a person or machine."[4] Data collection involves the observation and recording of events and transactions.

Data is not useful, however, until it is introduced to some form of processing to analyze and evaluate its significance. Data conversion then involves changing the data from its raw form into a more suitable form for processing and storage. Information is processed data that has been analyzed and evaluated to a point where it is meaningful and useful to the management information system (MIS) user.

There are many types of management information systems that range from simple to complex. The most basic system is a manual system. An example of a manual system is an occupational therapist recording muscle strength measurements on a manual muscle test form. The measurements are recorded on paper in numeric or alphabetic characters. The results of the test do not have meaning until the therapist evaluates and analyzes the measurements based on previous learning and knowledge.

Manual methods of collecting information are cumbersome, slow, and inefficient. Errors are likely to occur. It is difficult to use a manual method with increased volume demands or more complex requirements. Evaluation of the results of a single manual muscle test might be relatively straightforward. However, if the same therapist wanted to compare the results of a patient's/client's tests to the test results of other patients with the same diagnosis, it would be more difficult.

Another form of an information system is a mechanical system. Some examples of mechanical systems are typewriters, cash registers, and bookkeeping machines. Mechanical devices normally are used to make processing more rapid or legible than manual methods. These devices also enable the user to improve the accuracy of recording and calculating the data. Processing the information is not continuous. The recorded data must be transferred to another device for further analysis and evaluation.

An electro-mechanical information system is one in which data is converted from alphabetic or numeric characters, as in the manual and mechanical systems to punched holes to be read by electro-mechanical machines. Examples of this system are punched cards and paper tape that are fed into key punch machines to be interpreted. This system provides better speed and accuracy over the manual and mechanical methods. It is also very easy to store the data. However, one major problem is that the data is only in machine-readable form.

The most complex MIS is the electronic system. The electronic system requires that data be translated into magnetic and electronic impulses that are then acceptable to electronic devices, such as computers. Data is collected by many devices in many ways. Collection devices range from automatic devices, such as counters and sensors, to direct access drives, such as keyboards. The data is then stored and manipulated electronically with the resulting information in understandable form. Electronic systems are ideal for applications involving large amounts of data that must be collected, analyzed, and presented in an efficient and economic manner.

Electronic systems are the basis of today's computer information systems and the major focus of this chapter. Information systems can be defined as a network of computer-based data processing procedures that have been developed in an organized and integrated manner with manual systems for the purpose of providing timely, accurate and useful information to support decision making and other management functions.[11]

Why Do We Need Management Information Systems?

The first and most apparent need for a MIS is a limitation of the human mind to perceive and retain all the information it requires and to act on this information in a timely manner. Second, the social complexity of our environment has made it necessary to develop sophisticated techniques for handling data. No longer are simple explanations satisfactory to answer the complex curiosity of today's scholars. Third, there is a tremendous need to communicate the proliferation of new ideas and occupational therapy principles toward the end goal of improving the quality and sophistication of treatment of patients/clients.[4]

Information is power. The more accurate, timely, and complete our information, the better the quality of our decisions. Information that is not accurate is not helpful. The acronym GIGO, garbage in, garbage out, explains this issue. Information system or computer errors can usually be traced to incorrect input data or unreliable programs, both caused by human mistakes. Managers will always be held accountable for their actions that result from the decisions they make. The more information systems tend to reduce the uncertainty in decisions made by managers at all levels, the greater the value of the information.

Management information systems allow managers to process information with better accuracy, timeliness, completeness, and conscientiousness than they have ever been able to do in the past. This allows managers to be aware of problems and opportunities much faster. It enables them to devote more time to planning instead of manually analyzing results. It also permits managers to give timely consideration to more complex relationships and greatly assists in decision implementation. The MIS allows the collection of data in far greater quantities and combinations than before. It provides exceptional opportunities for evaluating products, business opportunities, customer and supplier relationships, as well as being a tremendous aid to decision making. Not only is more information able to be captured, but the quick manipulation and processing of that information gives managers capabilities to focus on relevant issues of the problem instead of concentrating on the data manipulation.

Management information systems are very powerful tools for managers. However, good information, produced by correct processing of accurate data is not enough by itself. Even good information must be coupled with a rational decision-making process. To aid decision making, the information system would provide the right information, to the right person, at the right time, in a cost-effective way.[8] The more closely the system is designed for the specific application of the user, the better the results. "Men will always be held accountable for the decisions they make. However, information systems will furnish men with the facts on which to base more effective and dependable decisions."[4]

What Are the Components of a Management Information System (MIS)?

There are three major components of a MIS system. They are:

- The users
- The hardware
- The software

The Users

As stated previously, a MIS provides the tools for manipulating data. However, the analysis of the data is the responsibility of the end user. Therefore a MIS must be designed with the users in mind. In designing systems we must move beyond just the technology and look at the social, psychological, and anthropolitical aspects of organizations and their specific relationship to the information system needed.[3] Systems must be designed to deal with human factors such as ease of use and understanding, compatibility with departmental functions, and other requirements of the particular situation. No matter how technologically advanced the system is, if the system designer has not gained the support of the users and the corporate culture, it is doomed to fail. People must recognize that a need or problem exists before they can develop a solution.

When implementing a MIS in an occupational therapy department, the staff must understand the benefits the system will have. Even a system as basic as word processing might be perceived as a threat to secretarial staff and as a criticism that their typing skills are not sufficient to meet departmental demands. Gaining their support, however, will make the implementation of a new system much easier and produce a more successful outcome.

The Hardware

Hardware involves two basic concepts—the machinery and the internal operations of the machine. Understanding the relationship between the two is necessary to conceptualize how the computer works. Each are discussed below.

In defining the basic components of computer hardware it is helpful to consider this analogy: The computer hardware is to software as a phonograph is to a record.

The physical equipment used for processing data into information is called hardware. This includes the computer as well as related components for data entry, storage, communication, and display. "A computer can be defined as a fast and accurate symbol or data manipulating system that is designed and organized to automatically accept and store input data, process them and produce output results under the direction of a detailed set of step-by-step program instructions."[11] The computer is not just used for computation, but is also an unequalled machine for data storage, retrieval, manipulation, and display. The computer uses electronic techniques to store, execute, and modify instructions that manipulate data in predefined ways. It is important to remember that although computers are excellent tools for processing transactions and as aids to decision making, they are unable to duplicate such human skills as creativity, pattern, recognition, intuitive reasoning, associate recall, and physical dexterity.[8]

There are four major classifications of computers: supercomputers, mainframes, minicomputers, and microcomputers. All types of computers have essentially the same kind of electronic circuitry and comprise similar elements of programming storage, input, and output. The differences of the four types of computers are based on size, speed, and applications.

Supercomputers are the largest, fastest, more expensive computers made. They are designed to process complex scientific applications, such as top secret weapons research for the federal government. The computational speed of the system is its most important feature.

Mainframe computers are one size below the supercomputers. They offer more speed and storage capacity than the minicomputer or microcomputer. They are able to handle large volumes of data, such as the information needs of an entire hospital. Mainframes have the ability to relay data to minicomputers and microcomputers at individual work stations through computer networks.

Minicomputers are the next smallest size. They are designed to handle the simultaneous processing needs of multiple users of microcomputers. There is considerable overlap between the most powerful microcomputers and the low end minicomputers. Minicomputers usually vary in size from a desk top model to the size of a small filing cabinet.

Microcomputers or personal computers (PCs) are the smallest computers that can execute program instructions to perform a wide variety of tasks. They are self contained units that are light enough to be moved around. They can be no larger than a hand held calculator or the size of a portable typewriter. PCs are designed to stand alone or as a single user system. There are two major types of microcomputers—those that have a hard disk drive capable of storing information directly in the computer or a two disk drive system that stores information on floppy disks. The development of microcomputers has revolutionized our ability to collect and analyze increasing amounts of information in occupational therapy departments.

There are many benefits of microcomputers to business as well as occupational therapy. The benefits stem from the quality of information or the extent of the usefulness of the information. The benefits increase with the timeliness, reliability, response time, completeness, and thoroughness of the information. The microcomputer allows us to gather information of greater quality in a more cost efficient manner. It provides us with increased capacity, more information, and more accurate results as well as permitting the introduction of new activities in a department, such as word processing or data management. It is also helpful in reducing staff and overcoming staffing shortages, such as secretarial staff.

Specific examples of benefits of microcomputers for occupational therapists are inventory management of activities of daily living supplies and word processing of home exercise or activity program instruction sheets. These applications and others will be discussed in the section on software.

The Central Processing Unit

The central processing unit (CPU) is the brain of the computer hardware. It is both the processor in which the instructions are executed and the main memory where instructions and data are stored. The function of the CPU is to select instructions, decode, and obey them. It controls the routing and processing of input and instructions.

There are three main sections of a CPU: the primary storage area, the arithmetic-logic section, and control section. The primary storage section contains four sections all relating to data being processed. There is an input storage area, where data is held until it is ready to be processed; a working storage area where data is held while it is being manipulated; an output storage area that holds the finished results of data manipulation; and a program storage area that holds the processing instructions. In addition to the primary storage or main memory section, most computers also have secondary or external storage capabilities, such as storage or magnetic disks or magnetic tape storage (Figure 2-1).

The arithmetic-logic section is where the actual data processing occurs. All mathematical calculations are made and all comparisons take place in this section. Once the calculations and comparisons are completed, the data is returned to the primary storage area.

The control section of the CPU coordinates all of these functions. The control section is responsible for selecting, interpreting, and implementing the execution of the program instructions. It directs the operation of the entire computer system. It is analogous to the central nervous system in the human body.

Figure 2-1
Components of Hardware

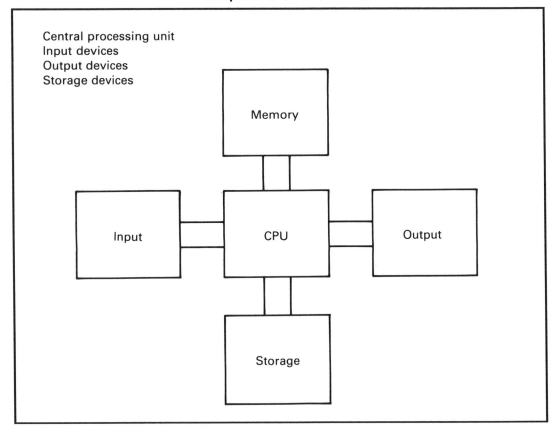

The main memory of the computer is in the CPU. The memory of the computer is made up of a series of microprocessor chips. The main memory is where data and instructions are stored until they are needed by the computer. The data in memory is stored in individual storage compartments. Each storage compartment has a unique numeric address, which is used to identify a particular storage location.

There are two major types of memory: read only memory (ROM) and random access memory (RAM). ROM holds permanent data programmed into the computer at the time of manufacture. It is not lost when the computer is turned off. ROM cannot and is not intended to receive data from the CPU. ROM holds short, start-up programs that give an immediate message to the user when turning on the machine and initiates the loading action of the operating system.[7]

RAM holds the software program and the dynamically changing data. Data and instructions are written, read, erased, and accessed randomly in this area. Random access implies that the data is accessed in a random method. It can be both read from and written to by the CPU. Data in RAM is lost when the computer is turned off. The size of RAM is what is referred to as the storage capacity of the computer. When the computer is initialized or turned on, the amount of RAM, such as 512K (kilobytes) is displayed on the screen. (See section on software.) The size of RAM dictates the speed and versatility of computer operations. Application programs will specify the minimum amount of RAM required for its use. Insufficient RAM will restrict the range of application programs.[7]

Input Devices

Input devices are necessary to enter and access information in the CPU. They allow some direct human/machine communication. In evaluating input devices, the closer to the source the data has been captured and the destination the output can be presented, the more effective the system. If data is captured the moment it arises and the output is presented directly in the form it is needed, the system should work in the fastest, most accurate, and cost efficient manner.[7] There are many types of input devices. The most common device is a visual display terminal (VDT). This consists of a terminal keyboard and display screen. The terminal keyboard is used to enter data into the CPU. A cathode ray tube, which looks like a television screen, is used to display the input data, receive messages, and process information from the computer.[9] The keyboard is used to enter user commands and data (comprised of numbers and text). It has two main functions—to act as a control console and accept input data. The keyboard has the conventional keys of a typewriter plus a special set of function keys.

Other input devices include a hand-held terminal, touchscreen, digipad, voice input, light pen devices, automatic reading devices, and modem. The hand-held terminal is a battery powered device comprised of a keypad, visual display, internal storage, data communication socket, and one or more stored programs. This terminal is initially connected to the computer either directly or via a telephone. A touchscreen allows the user to touch a point on the screen and the location of the screen is fed into the computer via an infrared grid. A light pen is also a device used to touch a screen to relay information to the computer. A digipad is a device that takes the form of a large tablet in which a light pen is moved over the tablet to trace out patterns on the pad, like an artist's palette.

A voice input device is a unit that is able to send commands to the computer via voice recognition. However, the unit must first be trained to recognize command words. A modem allows the input of data from one terminal to another, usually via the telephone. Automatic reading devices such as a wand or scanner are able to read information, such as universal product codes from food products in grocery stores.

Output Devices

Output devices are instruments of communication and interpretation between humans and the computer system. Output devices take results from the CPU and convert them into a form that can be understood and used by humans. Examples of output devices include printers, plotters, video display terminals, voice, and video monitors.

Printers accept a stream of electrical impulses from the computer and produce hard copy text or diagrams. Printers vary by the width of the print font or style, print quality, speed and volume. Laser printers are the fastest, most efficient and most expensive printers. Dot matrix printers, which produce a character image as a series of dots are fast, inexpensive, and produce good quality documents. Daisy wheel printers have a print head with 96 stems emanating from them like petals of a daisy. Each character is embossed on a small plate at the end of each stem. It has detachable printer heads to change the font or style of print. These are also very cost effective.

Printers allow processed information to be communicated by alpha-numeric text or in the form of graphs. Graphics can be in a monochrome, two dimensional display such as bar graphs or pie charts, or more refined and complex multicolor three dimensional pictures that can be used in computer aided design applications.[7]

Storage Devices

Storage devices are the means by which processed data is stored and then accessed at a future date. There is a hierarchy of storage devices. At the top of the storage hierarchy pyramid are the primary storage components found in the CPU. Next in line are the secondary or auxiliary storage elements. Many of these are direct access storage devices, such as hard disks or floppy disks. At the bottom of the pyramid are sequential access storage media that store data off line from the CPU. Examples of this include magnetic tape storage and punched paper media.

In microcomputers, direct access secondary storage is usually located on a hard disk or in floppy disks in the form of magnetic disks. In the hard disk system, 14 inch magnetic disks are permanently mounted in sealed contamination-free containers, in storage devices called disk drives. Smaller, floppy diskettes, which range from $3^1/2$ to 8 inches in diameter are a portable method of storage.

Software

Software is a set of programs, documents, and routines, associated with the operation of a computer system, that instructs the hardware what to do. A program can be defined as a detailed set of humanly prepared instructions that directs the computer to function in a specific way to produce a desired result. Programs can be plans to: achieve a solution to a problem, design, write, and test one or more routines, or with a set of sequenced instructions cause a computer to perform a particular operation.

There are four major levels of complexity in computer software. Each builds upon the capacities of the lowest level, the operating system. They are as follows:

- User-defined Fourth Generation Languages
- Packaged Programs
- Programming Languages
- Operating System

Operating System

Before we can use a computer's capacity to store and process data quickly and accurately, a suitable set of programs must be prepared to direct the computer's internal operation. This is called the operation system (OS). The operating system is an integrated set of programs that is used to manage the resources and overall operations of the computer. It is an organized collection of software that is designed to help the computer operators perform basic housekeeping tasks such as saving files, loading files, copying files and disks, formatting disks, and checking the status of the disk capacity.[11]

The operating system is the lowest level of software. It takes control of the computer as soon as it is turned on. The major objective of the operating system is to run the computer with a minimal amount of idle time during the processing of jobs. It is the program that directs all operations in the computer and determines the compatibility with different computers. The operating system is stored partly in ROM and partly on a disk, the disk operating system (DOS).

Programming Languages

Significant gains have been made in the development of software over the past 30 years. In the early 1950s, programmers had to write their problem solving instructions in special machine code numbers, called binary code, that computer circuits could understand. All computer programs are represented in binary codes.

The binary code involves the use of two symbols, 0 and 1. The data is relayed by a process of turning the 0 and 1 switches on and off. All words and numbers are represented in binary code.

An example of the relationship between the binary system and the decimal is as follows:[11]

Decimal	Binary
1	1
2	10
3	11
4	100
15	111
255	11111111

One binary code character is equal to a bit. A bit is defined as a physical component capable of storing exactly one of two possible conditions, the 0 and the 1. The term bit is formed from a contraction of the term *binary digit*. A byte is a group of 8 bits. A word then is a group of bytes treated as a unit. Four is the common number of bytes per word. A kilobyte is a thousand bytes or characters and a megabyte is a million bytes or characters.

Computer instructions usually occupy 4 to 24 bits and comprise 2 parts: an operation code and address. The operation code tells the computer what action it is to perform and the address tells the computer where it is stored.

Alphanumeric data is represented by binary code by a two stage conversion. First the character is expressed as a number, usually in American Standard Code for Information Interchange and then expressed in binary code as follows:

Alphanumeric	A
ASCII	65
Binary	1000001

As technology progressed, special programming languages were developed to permit the programmer to write instructions in a form easier for humans to understand. All programming languages consist of symbols, characters and usage rules that permit people to communicate with computers. Every language must have instructions that fall into the following categories:[11]

- Input/output instructions
- Calculation instructions
- Logic/comparison instructions
- Storage/retrieval and movement instructions

Some examples of well known programming languages include: *Beginners All-purpose Symbolic Instruction Code (BASIC)*, which is an interactive language that permits direct communication between user and computer system during the preparation and use of the program,[10] *Common Business Oriented Language (COBOL)*, which is used for business type data processing and *Formula Translator (FORTRAN)*, which services the needs of scientists, businesses, and statisticians for mathematical applications.[11]

With the introduction of programming languages, programmers were able to use the word "add" or the "+" symbol in place of the number 21. Unfortunately, the computer only recognized the number 21 as the mathematical instruction to add. Therefore, a translation program had to be developed that transforms the instructions prepared by people using a convenient language into the machine language codes required by the computer. Today, almost all problem solving programs are first written in languages preferred by people and then translated by special software or hardware into equivalent machine codes.[11]

Packaged Programs

The most common type of program today is called an application program. Most application programs are packaged programs. They are often written to control a particular task, such as sales accounting or stock recording. Other types of application programs are not designed for any particular system, but instead contain standard routines and a repertoire of commands that allow the user to create individual records and reports to meet specific needs. There are thousands of widely used application programs. Examples discussed later in the chapter include: data base management systems, word processing, and spreadsheets. The proliferation of application programs has greatly increased the acceptability and use of microcomputers.

User-defined Fourth Generation Languages

The highest levels of computer language are user-defined fourth generation languages. These give maximum flexibility to manipulate data at the time of use. An example of a fourth generation language would be an occupational therapist manipulating data on a personal computer from the hospital mainframe. Fourth generation languages are still in the development stage.

Most application programs are written on floppy disks. The information from these disks can be permanently stored on a hard disk drive or used in their portable state. The care of a floppy disk is critical to maintaining its life. It is important to keep floppy disks free and clear of dust and dirt, which can impair their storage capabilities.

What exactly is a floppy disk? A floppy disk is a thin film of mylar plastic that has a ferrous oxide coating and is in a lubricated plastic jacket. It works by magnetically storing ones and zeros in small areas, called tracks and sectors.[9] Tracks and sectors are a number of invisible concentric circles. The tracks and sectors are defined according to the operating system. Each disk has a spinning life of approximately 50 hours. One double sided diskette holds 368,640 bytes. One typed page equals 2500 bytes and one disk holds 148 pages.[9]

Application Programs

Word Processing

Word processing is defined as a program that allows the entry, editing, and manipulation of electronic data to create, view, edit, manipulate, transmit, store, retrieve, and print text. Word processing is a recognized productivity enhancer. It has revolutionized the efficiency and productivity of secretarial staff by eliminating the need for retyping an entire document each time corrections are made. At any time the original documents can be recalled and changes made. It enables the user to create document records ranging from simple memoranda or letters to full length reports and books, edit these records, and print them in the preferred format.[7] Word processing has also greatly improved the ability of occupational therapists to send personalized form letters to patients, modify exercise sheets to meet individual patient/client needs, quickly modify papers for publications, and prepare resumes. This entire book has been written with the assistance of a word processor.

Computers with word processing capabilities are often referred to as word processors. There are two types of word processors: dedicated word processors and microcomputer based word processors. Dedicated word processors are essentially sophisticated typewriters that have some computer capabilities. They are faster than microcomputer-based word processing systems, but are unable to perform any other applications. Microcomputer-based word processors utilize a program that runs specifically on a microcomputer for the purpose of word processing. Using a microcomputer gives the user the flexibility to also use the computer for other applications, such as database management or financial spreadsheets.

There are many features of a typical word processing program. The most basic feature of a word processing program is its ability to add, insert, move, and delete characters, words, lines, and areas of text on a screen without retyping the document. Another beneficial feature of a word processing program is that it allows the user to create a template for documents, such as form letters or contracts. A form letter can be merged with a list of names and addresses to print individualized and personalized letters. It is possible to automatically change dates and key phrases. If an occupational therapy department has a staff therapist position open, personalized letters could be sent to therapists in the area for purposes of recruitment.

The spellchecker or spell correction option is a feature that allows the user to correct misspelled words. The program contains a dictionary of commonly used words. It offers the user alternative spellings of words it does not recognize based on phonetics and typographical mishaps and then allows the replacement of a misspelled word automatically with a suggested alternative. The program also allows the operator to supply a substitute word or to determine that no correction is necessary.[5]

Other options include global search/replace where one word can be automatically replaced with another throughout the text. Word wrap allows the operator to continue typing without hitting return. The computer knows exactly how each line should be and moves an unfinished word to the next line. Margin justification allows straight right-hand margins by adding extra space called line filling. Pages can be automatically titled, the font and print style can be changed, and the title centered within a document. The user is able to set margins, tabs, and page lengths to meet specific individual needs.

Spreadsheets

Spreadsheets are financial modeling software. They are a series of grids on which financial statements, sales forecasts, budgets, and results of research studies can be built. Spreadsheets are the automated equivalent of accountants' multicolumn ledger sheets. Anything that lends itself to a grid or matrix organization can be set up in a spreadsheet format.

A spreadsheet manipulates numbers the way word processors manipulate words. It organizes data in a matrix of rows and columns, with each cell assigned a specific value or formula. Mathematical relationships can be set up between the cells. An example of this is:

Cell B12 = Cell A16 × Cell F50/Cell J30

Spreadsheets are very versatile tools for processing many numbers in a small amount of time. As discussed, cells are linked together by formulas. If you make a change in one cell, the spreadsheet uses the power of the computer to automatically recalculate and alter every other cell linked to the original cell.[1] Spreadsheets manipulate data according to the user's directions. They offer the four arithmetic functions, exponentiation, and rounding off, as well as summing a group of cells. Spreadsheets also calculate absolute values, averages, logarithms, and square roots. This application is extremely helpful for budgeting. Spreadsheets allow the manager to project different costs of supplies or salaries and evaluate the impact on the budget without doing multiple individual calculations on a calculator.

Spreadsheets take considerable time to set up. Initially, the worksheet must be laid out examining the relationship in the matrix. The tables and headings must be labeled as well as the formulas defined for the cells. Actual figures must be tested in the formulas to ensure that accurate results are being produced. Once tested, a template of the matrix can be saved on the disk and recalled for future use. The results of the spreadsheet can be printed in tables or in rudimentary bar graphs.

In evaluating spreadsheet software, it is important to make sure the software is compatible with the brand of computer you are using. The amount of RAM on the computer will determine how complex a software package will be able to be used on the system. As spreadsheet programs become more complex, they allow the integration of features found in word processing and data base management systems.

Data Base Management Systems

Data base management systems (DBMS) is a generalized program that allows the user to define the structure and content of files and update these files. DBMS is a system of collecting, organizing, and translating general data and information into a knowledge bank that can be applied to specific tasks and projects. It offers general facilities for creating computer records and retrieving information from them to produce general or selective reporting.

There are four major types of data base systems: list structures, hierarchical structures, network structures, and relational structures (Figure 2-2).

In list structures, records are linked together by pointers or arrows. These support many separate files, but only one can be accessed at a time. Hierarchical data bases are structured so that the relationship between the files and file data are fixed and inflexible. Data can be used within the structure, but the structure cannot be changed. Network data base structure permits the connection of files in a multidirectional manner. The most flexible data base is a relational data base structure. All relationships between the files and the file data are flexible. This type of software allows you to establish and change relationships at will. Any piece of data can be related to another.

To understand DBMS it is helpful to understand some common terms associated with it. There is a hierarchy of terms upon which all DBMS are designed. A character is a single character or symbol such as the letter A. A field is one or more characters treated as a unit. A record is one or more fields treated as a unit. A file is many records treated as a unit. The following example illustrates the hierarchy of the data base management terms:

Character = A
Field = First name, middle name, last name
Records = Full name and full address
File = Mailing list

The capabilities of DBMS are very extensive. The system enables the user to define and structure data into files and create and maintain the files by adding, deleting, or changing information. It also allows the user to select and sort specific data, to compare and analyze it, and to generate meaningful reports. As with spreadsheets the quality of the data base will depend on the time and care that goes into the data base design and preparation. Also, after the data entry items have been defined, the accuracy of the data entered must be verified. Inaccurate data is of little value. It is a waste of time to set up a data base unless you are willing to expend the time and effort to keep it accurate and up-to-date.[6]

Figure 2-2
Data Base Management Structures

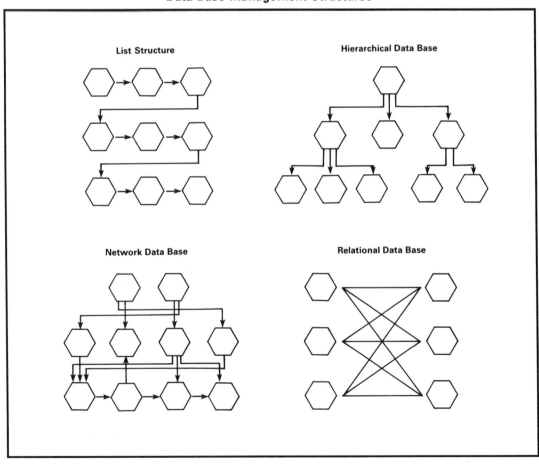

Questions

1. Management information systems:
   a. Are powerful tools for managers
   b. Can be as simple as transcribing data on a manual muscle test form
   c. A network of computer based data processing procedures that have been developed to provide timely, accurate, and useful information
   d. None of the above

2. Which of the following is not true about MIS?
   a. They allow managers to be aware of problems and opportunities faster
   b. They ensure that the data provided is accurate
   c. They give occupational therapists the ability to study and evaluate new treatment protocols
   d. They allow far greater quantities of data to be collected and analyzed

3. Which of the following is the least important element in MIS?
   a. Accurate information
   b. Rational decision making
   c. The support and cooperation of the users of the system
   d. A system that provides the right information to the right person at the right time

4. The central processing unit:
   a. Is the brain of the computer hardware
   b. Has three main sections: the primary storage section, the arithmetic-logic section, and the control section
   c. Contains two types of memory: RAM and ROM
   d. All of the above

5. Random access memory:
   a. Is not lost when the computer is turned off
   b. Holds the application programs and dynamically changing data
   c. Cannot receive information from the CPU
   d. None of the above

6. The operating system:
   a. Is the lowest level of software
   b. Is designed to help the computer perform basic housekeeping tasks
   c. Is a set of integrated programs that manage the overall operations of the computer
   d. All of the above

7. Word processing systems:
   a. Must be solely dedicated to performing only word processing functions
   b. On a microcomputer give the user flexibility for other software applications
   c. Are just glorified typewriters
   d. Are not cost or time efficient

8. Spreadsheet software:
    a. Is the automated equivalent of an accountant's multicolumn ledger sheet
    b. Is time consuming to set up
    c. Is a powerful tool for budget forecasting and research data analysis
    d. All of the above

9. Which of the following statements is not true?
    a. The least flexible data base system is a relational data base
    b. Hierarchical data bases have fixed relationships between files and file data
    c. List structures do not allow cross analyzing of data
    d. Network data bases permit the connection of files in a multidirectional manner

10. Data base management systems:
    a. Give the occupational therapist a meaningful structure in which to collect data
    b. Are of little value unless the data is accurate and up-to-date
    c. Gives the occupational therapist the ability to compare and analyze and then to produce meaningful reports
    d. All of the above

Answers
1. d
2. b
3. a
4. d
5. a
6. d
7. b
8. d
9. a
10. d

Case Study 1

The Department of Rehabilitation Services at Brigham and Women's Hospital, Boston, Massachusetts was having trouble maintaining sufficient quantities of ADL supplies in the department. There were frequent stockouts of commonly used items, such as long handled sponges and shoe horns. Another problem was that large quantities of special supplies were ordered and used by only a few patients. Consequently, many items in the ADL supply closet were obsolete. Running out of supplies caused frustrations for the occupational therapists and the patients. This lack of supplies did not allow the OTRs to provide optimum quality of care. It was very costly to the department to carry large amounts of excess inventory.

To solve the problem, a formalized inventory system needed to be developed that accounted for weekly/monthly usage of items in the department to provide a sufficient supply to prevent stockouts. To accomplish this task, the managers and coordinators met to discuss the problem and to suggest ideas to resolve it. A successful information system on inventory requires gaining support of the users to acknowledge a need for change and make sure it meets their needs.

The first step in the process was to take a manual count of all ADL supplies—the quantity and variety—in the department to determine which were still relevant and then prepare an inventory supply list. The next step was to evaluate the amount of supplies used each week and the time it takes to order and receive supplies. Next, quantity discounts were explored and a reorder quantity and reorder point were developed for each inventory item. The reorder point is a trigger point that indicates that it is time to place an order when a given quantity of supplies remain in stock.

Once this information was gathered, the inventory system was ready to be computerized. A data base management software program was chosen to allow development of records on each item in stock and specific vendors that supplied the products. Files were developed on all products and vendors. An example of a product record is:

PRODUCT RECORD

Product Name:	Elastic Laces
Product Number:	1443
Vendor:	Alimed
Unit Discount:	N/A
Unit Cost:	$.25
Monthly Usage:	150
Order Amount:	200
Reorder Point:	50

This record is part of a product file on all ADL equipment related to personal care. The product files were then grouped together with the vendor files to complete the data base.

The data base was set up as a relational data base. This allowed reports to be generated that cross-referenced different files. A report often generated was the list of vendor names and addresses with the product name, number, and order amount. This served as a useful reference to the secretary ordering the supplies.

The inventory system saved the Department of Rehabilitation Services $3,000 its first year. It also reduced the number of stockouts by 20% and saved time ordering. Most importantly, the quality of patient/client care was improved.

Case Study 2

Occupational therapists working in rehabilitation units of hospitals must often design home exercise or activity programs for their patients/clients prior to discharge. Designing and writing these programs to personalize them to meet the individual needs of the patient/clients is often a time consuming and tedious process. For certain diagnoses, such as total hip replacements, the programs for different patients/clients are often similar. To reduce the time of individual occupational therapists writing numerous home programs, this information is being computerized using word processing software.

Dewey Rehabilitation Hospital has instituted such an information system. To start the process, a group of occupational therapists met to discuss the value of such an information system and how it could increase their time to do more active therapy with the patients/clients. Their first step was to list all the necessary components of a complete home program. Individual occupational therapists were asked to develop sample home programs related to common patient/client needs, such as self range of motion exercises, energy conservation techniques, architectural barriers, and safety. Each individual occupational therapist's program was typed on the word processor to facilitate modifications. The occupational therapists then met as a group to review and discuss each other's proposals.

Once the group agreed upon the content of each subject area, the information was finalized on the word processor. A program was designed to allow the individual therapist to pick and choose what information would be given the patient/client. All the therapist had to do was select the topic relevant to patient/client, such as safety in the home, and print out the items, such as bathroom safety. The therapist was also able to personalize the home program by printing the patient's/client's name and address at the top. The program allowed the occupational therapist to add specialized instructions as necessary.

The therapists were extremely happy with the success of their efforts. The information system they developed allowed them to produce a professional, personalized home activity program in a short period of time. The system was flexible to meet individual patient/client needs, and was very time and cost effective. The information contained in the program could be updated quickly and easily on the word processor.

References

1. Ahl DH. What is a Spreadsheet? *Creative Computing.* 10:6(51)513, 1984.
2. Bruns WJ, McFarlan FW. *How Information Technology is Changing Management Control Systems.* Harvard Business School, 1987.
3. Burch JG. Designing Information Systems for People. *J. Sys. Manag.* 37:10(30)33, 1986.
4. Dipple G, House WC. *Information Systems: Data Processing and Evaluation.* Glenview, Ill: Scott, Foresman, 1969.
5. Fleming MV. Micros and Word Processing in the Automated Office. *The Office* 104:5(118)127, 1986.
6. Jacobson B. What is a Data Base Package? *Creative Computing* 10:9(51)511, 1984.
7. Longley D, Shain M. *The Microcomputer Users Handbook.* New York: Wiley, 1984.
8. Mader C. *Information Systems: Technology, Economics, Application, Management.* Chicago: Science Research Associates, 1979.
9. *Personal Computer Training.* Boston: First Micro Group. 1985.
10. Sage D. Electronic Spreadsheet: A Versatile Tool. *Forest Industries.* 112:1(40)41, 1985.
11. Sanders DH. *Computers Today.* New York: McGraw-Hill, 1983.

CHAPTER 3

Marketing Occupational Therapy Services

Karen Jacobs, EdD, OTR/L, FAOTA

Introduction

> . . .We are on the verge of an era when the needs for our services are so great as to push us to the brink of glory, if we can only deliver; or we may stumble, because we shall, I fear, cling tenaciously to what we have done without looking at what we might do if we were to take bold new directions.[6]

These were the words spoken by Cromwell in 1968. If the concept of marketing had been applied to the profession of occupational therapy 20 years ago, just imagine how much more of a significant role we may have been playing in the health care marketplace today.

The need for occupational therapy practitioners to have a good understanding of and apply the concepts of marketing has become more critical today. Marketing can play an important part in the success of an occupational therapy program and should become a familiar framework for the occupational therapy manager.

What is Marketing?

Marketing has been a misunderstood term, most often used synonymously with public relations, selling, fundraising, or development. However, according to marketer Peter Drucker, "the aim of marketing is to make selling superfluous."

"Marketing consists of meeting peoples' needs in the most efficient and therefore profitable manner."[16] Kotler and Clarke define marketing in the following manner:

> **Marketing** is the analysis, planning, implementation, and control of carefully formulated programs designed to bring about voluntary exchanges of values

with target markets for the purpose of achieving organizational objectives. It relies heavily on designing the organization's offering in terms of the target markets' needs and desires, and on using effective pricing, communication, and distribution to inform, motivate, and service the markets.[11]

Successful marketing planning begins with an idea that serves as the framework for all marketing efforts. It is an orientation that makes satisfying the customer's needs the integrating organizational principle. While the first impulse of the marketing novice is to design a program, such as a school-based work-related occupational therapy program and then look for customers, for example adolescents with developmental disabilities, effective marketing dictates that the process be reversed. One first looks at the market and listens carefully to potential customers and then designs the program to match the needs and desires of these potential customers.

Marketing Planning

The main benefits of marketing planning can be summarized as follows:

1. Encourages systematic thinking ahead by management
2. Leads to better coordination of organizational efforts
3. Leads to the development of performance standards for control
4. Causes the organization to sharpen its guiding objectives and policies
5. Results in better preparedness for sudden developments
6. Brings about a more vivid sense in the participating managers of their interacting responsibilities[3]

Marketing planning can be viewed as a three-step process. Figure 3-1 delineates this process with planning as the first step. It encompasses identifying attractive markets, developing marketing strategies and developing action programs. Execution is the second step. It includes carrying out the action programs. Finally the third step involves marketing control. This final step requires measuring results, analyzing the causes of poor results, and taking corrective action. Adjustments in the plan, its execution, or both would include corrective actions that could be implemented.

Identifying Attractive Target Markets

Identifying the demands of the market is the first step in marketing. The market is defined as all actual or potential buyers of a product, service or idea and can be considered in its entirety, such as all referral sources to an early intervention program or divided into relevant segments according to variables such as types of professionals, for example physicians, special education teachers, or nurses. Identifying attractive target markets includes the analysis of marketing opportunities.

This analysis consists of:

1. A self-audit
2. Consumer analysis
3. An analysis of other providers of similar services
4. An environmental assessment

Self-Audit

A self-audit assesses the strengths, weaknesses, opportunities, and threats (SWOT Analysis) of your department and/or specific program. Factors to be assessed may include:

1. The reputation of your facility in the community
2. The staff and their qualifications, such as a master's degree, certification as a hand therapist or specialized training, e.g. NDT
3. Physical size of the program
4. Location of the program, for example hospital/rehabilitation setting, community-based
5. Convenience of your location to mass transit, highways and parking
6. Type and quality of equipment
7. Available budget
8. Support from administration

Figure 3-1
The Marketing Planning and Control System

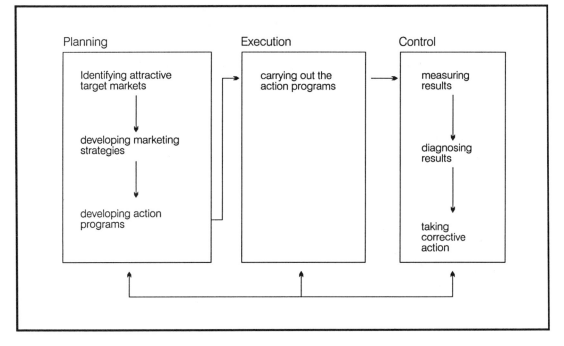

This self-audit assists in understanding how well or poorly prepared you are to meet the marketplace demands. Ascertaining what you do well and maintaining that product (service) at an optimal level is part of marketing.

Consumer Analysis

It is important to assess the potential consumers of your occupational therapy department's services within your catchment area. An analysis of some of the consumers who might use your products may include:

1. Physicians
2. Nurses
3. Special education teachers
4. Administrators
5. Social workers
6. Insurance companies
7. Rehabilitation managers and consultants
8. Vocational counselors
9. Attorneys
10. Injured workers
11. Industrial companies
12. Colleagues, such as other OTs, COTAs, PTs

Analysis of Other Providers of Similar Services

How adequately the needs of the marketplace are being met, what areas are not being served, where duplication and overlap are occurring, and where opportunities for collaboration or joint venture exist can be ascertained through an analysis of other providers of similar services. One simple way to obtain information is to place your name on the mailing list of facilities/companies providing a similar product line. Reading through newsletters, brochures, etc. from the competition can be very insightful!

Environmental Assessment

The changes and trends that may have an impact on occupational therapy services and perhaps the future of the profession compose an environmental assessment. These include:

1. Demographic Variables
2. Political and Regulatory Systems
3. Cultural Environment
4. Economic/Financial Environment
5. Psychographics
6. Technological Developments

Demographics

Demographics is the study of human populations according to such variables as age, sex, family size, family life cycle, income, occupation, education, religion, race, and nationality. For example, the increasing number of elderly individuals is a demographic trend that should have an impact on occupational therapy services.

Political and Regulatory Systems

Both political and regulatory systems may have an impact on occupational therapy services. For example, those occupational therapy programs located in the states of Florida, Ohio and Kentucky who are interested in developing work hardening programs will find that to receive reimbursement through their Workers' Compensation system they will need to become accredited by the regulatory agency, the Commission on Accreditation of Rehabilitation Facilities (CARF), and adhere to CARF's Work Hardening Guidelines.[5,7]

The implementation of the Americans With Disabilities Act (ADA) can have importance to the occupational therapy profession. Occupational therapy practitioners can be advocates and assist in implementing the ADA which provides comprehensive civil rights protections from discrimination in employment, transportation, public accommodations, telecommunications, and the activities of state and local government for individuals with disabilities. For example, Title 1—Employment provides the occupational therapist with the opportunity to provide post-offer screenings and devise reasonable accommodations so that the individual with a disability can perform the essential functions of the job.[1]

Cultural Environment

Culture is a force that affects individuals within society's behaviors, values, perceptions, preferences and behaviors. The United States is becoming a more multicultural society; and it becomes imperative that occupational therapy practitioners develop an understanding and sensitivity to the culture profiles of clients within their catchment area. Having practitioners who are bilingual can be most beneficial and may be the variable that assists in making a product successful.

Economic/Financial Environment

An analysis of the economic/financial environment revealed that the following factors may have a positive impact for occupational therapy services:

a. Eight percent of the gross national product is spent on programs that support dependency.
b. One in five American adults suffers from some type of disability.
c. Over $45 billion a year is spent on Workers' Compensation.
d. Ten percent of corporation expenditures are spent on health care.
e. Approximately 300,000 students with disabilities who graduate each year from high schools are unemployed.[8]

Psychographics

Psychographics is the technique of measuring consumer's social class, lifestyle and personality characteristics and can provide information on activities, interests and opinions of these individuals. Understanding the psychographic profile of your consumer might provide information to assist in strategizing a product to them.

Technological Developments

The technology arena is greatly advancing and will have an impact on the type of "high tech" evaluation and treatment equipment available to occupational therapy programs. As computers become more commonplace in occupational therapy departments, these technological advances will allow for information to be exchanged in a more efficient manner. For example, many programs send instantaneous reports to insurance companies within 24 hours via a computer modem or communicate worldwide in a matter of seconds through a facsimile machine.

Selecting Target Markets & Market Segments

Once analysis is completed, there are three steps in target marketing:

Market segmentation refers to the act of dividing a market into distinct groups of buyers who might require separate products and marketing mixes. For example, physicians can be segmented into pediatricians or neurologists; allied health professionals can be segmented into speech pathologists and physical therapists.

Market targeting is the act of evaluating and selecting one or more of the markets to enter. An example of this is targeting orthopedic surgeons as the main referral source for a hand therapy program.

Product positioning is the act of formulating a competitive position for the product and a detailed marketing mix.

Developing Marketing Strategies

Developing marketing strategies includes the development of objectives for each identified target market and their implementation. The four P's—product, place, price and promotion are the strategies that can be used to influence the demand for a product. Here is how each of these "P's" is used is the marketing mix.[4,10]

Product

Simply stated, what we do as occupational therapy practitioners are our products. That is, occupational therapy assists individuals to become as independent as possible.

Ideally, the goal is to offer a product line, that is, a variety of products associated with one another by a overall theme. For example, an occupational therapy department may have an industrial rehabilitation program whose product line includes: post-offer screening, baseline evaluation, job capacity evaluation, occupational capacity evaluation, work capacity evaluation, ergonomic consultation, and work hardening; whereas a school-based occupational therapy department may offer a product line of sensory integration evaluation and treatment, work-related assessment and programming and classroom consultation.

How a product is packaged may influence its success. It is important to make sure all your paperwork, for example, brochures and evaluation write-ups have a professional appearance. The ability to access information quickly and be able to present it in a professional manner to the target markets is an asset.

Many new product ideas are generated by understanding our client's needs and wants through direct surveys, projective tests, focus group discussions, and letters and complaints received. It is important to note that for every unhappy customer, you lose 50 others; and that 80% of your business is coming from 20% of your customers.[2]

Place
Occupational therapy services can be provided in a variety of places. Some of these include:

1. Free standing facilities located in professional buildings, industrial parks, and shopping centers
2. Free standing facility affiliated with outpatient service departments, rehabilitation centers or hospitals
3. As part of a comprehensive rehabilitation or acute care facility/program/hospital
4. At work site programs provided by a company to serve the needs of a specific business or industry
5. Schools
6. Nursing homes

When analyzing the *place* aspect of marketing planning, other variables that should be considered are the hours the program is offered for business. For example, is your program open during hours convenient to your market(s) or your staff? An innovative aspect of place could be the provision of day care services for the children and/or elderly patients of clients who are attending your program.

Price
The price or fee schedule for occupational therapy services (products) should be based on cost, competitive factors, geographic area, and what the consumer is willing to pay. It is important for the price to be commensurate with perceived value.[10]

Promotion
Promotion is the vehicle of communicating information to your markets about the product's merits, place and price. Instruments of promotion are: advertising, sales promotion, publicity, and personal selling.

Advertising
Advertising involves the use of a paid message presented in a recognized medium and by an identified sponsor, with the purpose to inform, persuade, and remind.

Some advertising vehicles include:

Printed ads—found in newspapers, journals and magazines

Brochures

Direct mail

Broadcasts

Transits

Billboards

Quarterly newsletter

Sales Promotion

Sales promotion is the use of a wide variety of short-term incentives to encourage purchase of the product. This approach is most effective when used in conjunction with advertising. For example, at an open house for an industrial rehabilitation program a successful sales promotion technique used to increase new referrals was a business card drawing for "service certificates" good for a day's worth of work hardening or work evaluation on any new referrals.

Publicity

"Publicity is often described as a marketing stepchild because it is relatively underused in relation to the real contribution it can make."[13] The most positive aspect of publicity is that it is free. However, one has little control over the placement of it and thus it becomes difficult to focus publicity on specific target markets. An example of publicity might be to contact the local media, through a press release, about an upcoming event at your facility, e.g. activities to celebrate occupational therapy month. Perhaps if the media finds your event newsworthy and they are not understaffed, they will send a reporter to cover the event. Whether or not the reporter writes a story can be dependent on variables out of your control, such as available time and space in the newspaper. However, a successful strategy in utilizing publicity more effectively has been to develop a rapport with the media. Personally contact your local newspaper and radio station and introduce yourself, let them know about your program and offer to be available to them if they need a resource.

Personal Selling

Face-to-face communication between you and your audience is the most effective form of promotion. It is, however, the most expensive. It is also the method most used by occupational therapy practitioners.[10] Word of mouth recommendations by staff and consumers of an occupational therapy program (products) are a powerful sales pitch. Other successful personal selling methods include the following:

Exhibiting at various conferences

Developing a free speakers' bureau

Presenting inservice training to physicians and occupational and physical therapy practitioners

Presenting continuing education workshops

Lecturing

Attending professional meetings for various organizations
Holding an open house
Holding continuing education seminars for referral sources

Focus groups have been found to be an effective marketing technique. These techniques use primary referral sources, such as physicians, to provide feedback on current programming efforts and recommendations for future program modifications. The use of focus groups allows the manager to quickly incorporate modifications perceived to be important by the referral sources. This in turn should generate an increased commitment on the part of the referral sources to the program.

Focus Group Interviewing

"Focus group interviewing is becoming one of the major marketing research tools for gaining insight into consumer thoughts and feelings."[12] Focus group interviewing consists of inviting six to ten participants to spend a few hours with a *skilled* interviewer to discuss any designated subject matter, such as the feasibility of developing a school-based occupational therapy work program.

Focus group practitioners are usually paid a small sum for attending the meeting. These are typically held in pleasant surroundings, with refreshment served. The interview begins with broad questions, such as "What do you think about occupational therapy work programming for elementary school-aged special needs students?" Leading to "focusing" in on more specific questions on the subject matter such as "What do you think about the feasibility of an occupational therapy work program being established at Butler Elementary School?" "The interviewer encourages free and easy discussion among participants, hoping that the group dynamics will bring out deep feelings and thoughts."[14] Although the results cannot be generalizable to the market as a whole due to its small sample size, the information gathered can provide insight into participants' perceptions, attitudes and satisfaction. Information obtained can help define what issues need to be researched more formally or may provide the foundation for being able to develop a product which will meet the consumer's needs.[14]

Execution of the Marketing Plan

Once you have selected your target market, develop a specific marketing mix (product, price, place and promotion) for your market which stresses the benefits of your product(s). When executing action programs a time line should be delineated, such as a 12 month period, to measure whether objectives and goals are being met. The action plan should be dynamic and be able to be changed throughout the year as new opportunities and problems arise. Ideally, actions should be assigned to specific individuals who are given exact completion dates. An action that might be assigned to a staff therapist can include developing a single paragraph description of the sensory integration program provided by the occupational therapy department. The therapist is given a one week time line to complete this action. Once the description is completed, the manager has two weeks to incorporate this information into a brochure being developed to promote the expanded product line of pediatric occupational therapy to potential referral sources. In this case, as in all aspects of promotion, it is important to communicate in a language that is familiar to your market. Avoid professional jargon!

Marketing Control

"Marketing is an area where rapid obsolescence of objectives, policies, strategies, and programs is a constant possibility."[14] Marketing control attempts to circumvent this dilemma and assist in maximizing the probability that a product will achieve its short- and long-term objectives.

It is important to measure program results, diagnose these results and take corrective action, if necessary. There are three types of marketing control:

1. **Annual plan control** consists of the steps used during the year to monitor and correct deviations from the marketing plan to assure that annual sales and profit goals are being achieved.
2. **Profitability control** refers to the efforts used to determine the actual profit or loss of different marketing entities such as the products (services) or market segments.
3. **Strategic control** is a systematic evaluation of the organization's market performance in relation to the current and forecasted marketing environment.[14]

Unfortunately, as uncommon as marketing planning is in health care organizations, marketing control is even less common. If health care organizations do bother to evaluate performance, it is usually limited to clinical evaluation: 'We provided a (clinically) good service.' In the process of providing these services, however, health care organizations are often squandering scarce resources, unaware of which resources are being productively used and which are being wasted.[14]

Conclusion

A bright future can be a certainty for therapists who are prepared to accept the reality of today's and tomorrow's health care environment. It will be increasingly competitive, with various professions vying for control of the patient and, thereby, the dollars. It will be increasingly complex. It will be increasingly controlled by payors—government, insurers, and corporations.[19]

Therapists' abilities to market—yes, market!—their skills and knowledge to those that control the dollars will be an ever-present requirement for success. It will likely make the difference between encroachment by other professions and a resulting second-class specialty, and a proud and effective profession placed squarely in a leadership position within the health care industry.[19]

We need to rally to this cheer! Marketing should guide the occupational therapy practitioner in his or her role as a manager in the marketplace. Having access to an expert in marketing to assist in the development of a marketing plan would be the ideal situation, but this is not always the case. On the other hand, the worst possible scenario would be one where even an informal market analysis does not precede program development. If this is the case for you, a word of caution. Remember that designing a program and then looking for customers typically leads to facing an uphill battle to success. At the very least, before investing a great deal of useless time, effort and money, attempt to perform a market analysis on your own following the guidelines presented in this chapter and in other available literature.

Questions

1. Peter Drucker describes the aim of marketing as:
   a. Making selling superfluous
   b. Maximizing sales
   c. Obtaining the highest price on your product
   d. Developing the largest size product line

2. A market is:
   a. All actual or potential buyers of a product, service or idea
   b. A place
   c. A price
   d. Transactions between two buyers of a product

3. The technique of interviewing a selected group of individuals is called:
   a. Task group interviewing
   b. Activity analysis
   c. Strategic marketing interviewing
   d. Focus group interviewing

4. Which of the following is a false statement regarding the benefits of marketing planning?
   a. Encourages systematic thinking
   b. Results in better preparedness for sudden development
   c. Leads to better coordination of an organization's efforts
   d. Leads to the development of poorer performance standards for control

5. An individual's lifestyle is measured by the technique called:
   a. Cognitive analysis
   b. Psychographics
   c. Life cycle analysis
   d. Lifestyle

6. The most common promotion technique used by occupational therapists is:
   a. Advertising
   b. Personal selling
   c. Sales promotion
   d. Publicity

7. What is not a type of marketing control?
   a. Annual plan control
   b. Profitability control
   c. Strategic control
   d. Segment marketing control

8. Which are the three steps in target marketing?
    a. Market segmentation, market targeting, product positioning
    b. Market segmentation, market targeting, price positioning
    c. Product positioning, price targeting, market segmentation
    d. Market targeting, market pricing, target place

9. The four P's of marketing mix are:
    a. Price, packaging, place, promotion
    b. Place, price, promotion, product
    c. Product, packaging, promotion, place
    d. Product, procedure, price, packaging

10. The three-step process for marketing planning and control is:
    a. Planning—execution—control
    b. Control—execution—planning
    c. Execution—planning—control
    d. Planning—control—execution

Answers
1. a
2. a
3. d
4. d
5. b
6. b
7. d
8. a
9. b
10. a

Case Study 1

The sole occupational therapist in a private school for learning disabled students ages 5 to 21 wants to expand her product line to include work assessment and programming.

After approaching the school's administrator about this idea, she is told that she must first develop a marketing plan to support the feasibility of such a venture.

The therapist approached this task as a three-step process: planning, execution, and control.

Step One—Planning

Within *planning* there are three steps: identifying attractive markets, developing marketing strategies and developing action programs.

The first step was to identify target markets and consisted of:

- A self-audit
- Consumer analysis
- An analysis of other providers of similar services
- An environmental assessment

Self-Audit. In performing a self-audit the following strengths were revealed: there was both physical space for expansion of the program and enough funds for the purchase of specialized supplies and equipment, and the occupational therapist had an excellent reputation within the school.

Consumer Analysis. Although the therapist wanted to provide work assessment and programming to the complete student market, she narrowed her focus and targeted those learning disabled students ages 12 to 21 years.

Other Providers of Similar Services. There were no other providers of similar services; however, academic programming utilized a functional curriculum approach that might provide the opportunity for future collaboration.

Environmental Assessment. The catchment area for the school was 80 communities providing for a large cross-section of students. In addition, the school itself was located in an upper-middle class community among many service industries.

Marketing Strategies. The four P's - product, price, place, and promotion were analyzed as follows:

Product Line—Work assessments, work programming, classroom consultation to teachers

Price—The charge for occupational therapy already has been incorporated into the total school tuition

Place—Programming will be located in various areas: local stores, classrooms, school cafeterias and occupational therapy treatment areas

Promotion—The therapist will provide inservice training to teachers on the programming, devise a display for the school corridor with photographs of students in work occupational therapy, and contact a local newspaper to write an article about the program.

Step Two—Execution

Step Three—Control

Once the program has been executed, the third step will be to monitor whether the program is meeting its goal and objectives. This would be a dynamic process, where changes would be made and the three-step process would begin again.

Case Study 2

There are seven occupational therapists in a hand therapy clinic that is part of and located in an acute care hospital. Industrial rehabilitation, particularly work hardening, have become the new 'buzz words' in occupational therapy and the occupational therapy department would like to begin to include this aspect of practice into its product line.

As director of the occupational therapy department, you decide to perform a market analysis to ascertain the feasibility of expanding your product line to include industrial rehabilitation.

Your first step is to identify attractive target markets. In identifying these markets, the analysis of marketing opportunities should be performed. In this case the analysis consists of:

- A self-audit
- Consumer analysis
- An analysis of other providers of similar services
- An environmental assessment

A self-audit of the occupational therapy department consists of analyzing its strengths, weaknesses, opportunities and threats (SWOT analysis). For example, some strengths might include:

- Seven master's degree level occupational therapists. Three of these therapists have specialized training and certification as hand therapists
- Both the hospital and the occupational therapy department have an excellent reputation in the community
- The hospital is conveniently located near mass transit and major highways, and has attached parking

The analysis might reveal the following weaknesses:

- Limited physical space within the department for expansion
- Limited financial resources for the purchase of new equipment

The following opportunities might be revealed:

- The hospital recently purchased an office building in close proximity to the hospital and all available space has not been allocated
- Funding would be available for programs being housed in this new facility

At present, the aspect thought to be a threat is that the available space in the new freestanding facility would be assigned to a department other than occupational therapy.

A *consumer analysis* reveals the following markets as potential users of the industrial rehabilitation program:

- Physicians
- Nurses
- Insurance companies
- Attorneys
- Injured workers
- Local industry
- Rehabilitation managers and consultants
- Colleagues, such as other occupational therapists

An analysis of other providers of similar services revealed that there were no industrial rehabilitation programs in any other acute care hospital or outpatient rehabilitation facility within a 30-mile radius of the hospital.

Finally, an *environmental assessment* indicated that the hospital was located in a lower-middle class, blue collar community, with construction being the predominate industry.

Once the analysis was completed, *market segmentation* was performed. That is, the potential consumers of the industrial rehabilitation program were divided into distinct groups. For example, physician were segmented into orthopedic surgeons and neurologists. This market was targeted further by selecting only the orthopedic surgeons as the main referral source for the industrial rehabilitation program.

Developing marketing strategies specific to each targeted market is the next step in the analysis. In this case, the director decided to start with the orthopedic surgeons as the primary market. At this point, the director enlisted the assistance of the hospital's marketing department. Working together, they devised the four P's. The *product*, an industrial rehabilitation program, was divided into a product line that included: work capacity evaluation, work hardening, job analysis, and preplacement screening. The industrial rehabilitation program would be located (the *place*) in the newly acquired freestanding office building owned by the hospital. The *price* for the program would continue to be regulated by the hospital's fee schedule. *Promotion* was handled through the marketing department of the hospital, who would *advertise* the industrial rehabilitation program in the orthopedic surgeon's quarterly newsletter, and in its monthly professional journal, develop brochures and send direct mailings to these physicians. The *publicity* used to promote the industrial rehabilitation program to orthopedic surgeons would be through articles in the hospital's monthly newsletter and human interest stories that would focus on an individual client's successful return to work. Additional stories could be covered by the local community newpaper. Finally, the occupational therapists would become directly involved with *personal selling* by holding an open house for the orthopedic surgeons and providing a presentation of the industial rehabilitation program at the monthly physician's breakfast.

Once the industrial rehabilitation program was in place, it would be analyzed on a six-month basis to determine that program goals and objectives were being met.

References

1. Americans With Disabilities Act. Federal Register. July 26, 1991.
2. Baum, C.M. & Luebben, A.J. (1986). *Prospective Payment Systems: A Handbook for Health Care Clinicians.* Thorofare, NJ: SLACK Inc.
3. Branch, M. (1962). *The Corporate Planning Process.* New York: American Management Association.
4. Clopton, D. (1986, May 14). Marketing occupational therapy. *Occupational Therapy Forum,* pp. 15, 19.
5. Commission on Accreditation of Rehabilitation Facilities: 1991 Edition of the Standards Manual for Organizations Serving People with Disabilities. (1991). Tucson: Commission on Accreditation of Rehabilitation Facilities.
6. Cromwell, F. AOTA, 1968.
7. Ellexson, M. (1989). Work hardening. In Work programs guidelines. Rockville, MD: American Occupational Therapy Association.
8. Gilfoyle urges promotion of OT during AOTA conference ceremony. (1988, August 22). *OT Week,* p. 1 & 31.
9. Hershman, A.G. (1984). Reimbursement in private practice. *American Journal of Occupational Therapy,* 38(5), 299-306.
10. Jacobs, K. (May, 1987). Marketing occupational therapy. *American Journal of Occupational Therapy,* 41(5), 315-320.
11. Kotler, P. & Clarke, R. (1987). *Marketing for health care organizations.* Englewood Cliffs, NJ: Prentice-Hall.
12. Kotler, P. (1983a). *Principles of Marketing.* (2nd ed.). Englewood Cliffs, NJ: Prentice-Hall.
13. Kotler, P. (1983b). *Principles of Marketing—Instructor's Manual with Cases.* Englewood Cliffs, NJ: Prentice-Hall.
14. Kotler, P. & Clarke, R. (1984). *Marketing Management.* (5th ed.). Englewood Cliffs, NJ: Prentice-Hall.
15. LaCroix, E. (1987, October 30). *Setting Up and Surviving a Private Practice.* Bedford, MA: Massachusetts Association for Occupational Therapy Annual Conference.
16. Marketing occupational therapy services. (1984, August). *Occupational Therapy Newspaper,* p. 4.
17. Occupational therapy benefits from CARF changes. (1987). *Occupational Therapy News,* 41, 1.
18. Olson, T. & Urban, C. (1985). Marketing. In J. Bair & M. Gray (Eds.). *The Occupational Therapy Manager.* Rockville, MD: The American Occupational Therapy Association.
19. Pickelle, C. & Ramos, T. Publishers' Message. *Rehab Management,* February/March, 1991, p. 9.
20. Richardson, J.E. (1987). (Ed.) *Marketing 87/88.* Gullford, Conn: The Dushkin Publishing Group, Inc.
21. Scott, S. & Dennis D. (1988). (Eds.) *Payment for occupational Therapy Services.* Rockville, MD: The American Occupational Therapy Association.

CHAPTER 4

Ethical Issues in Occupational Therapy

Gail M. Bloom, MA, OTR/L

Introduction

A clear understanding of ethics is essential to obtaining a professional mastery of occupational therapy. The foundations of occupational therapy are linked with value-based concepts such as quality of life, competency, autonomy, self-determination, justice, and duty, necessitating that the occupational therapist acquire a systematic understanding of the profession's underlying values and basic moral beliefs.

The Importance of Ethics

Ethics is the branch of philosophy that concerns itself with morality. Within the domain of ethics are questions of right versus wrong, justice, equality, free will, and responsibility.

In 399 B.C., the people of ancient Athens condemned to death the father of moral philosophy, Socrates. His student, Plato, documented and elaborated on the thoughts of Socrates in his work, *The Republic*. In turn, Aristotle was a student of Plato and these three great thinkers provided the foundation for Western philosophical thought. The great issues debated at the origins of Western philosophy are still alive in the current attempts to develop an ethical framework for decision making. In the centuries following Socrates, Plato, and Aristotle, ethical inquiry was expanded most prominently by the works of St. Thomas Aquinas, St. Augustine, Jeremy Bentham, Thomas Hobbes, Immanual Kant, John Locke, John Stuart Mill, and Bertrand Russell.

In essence, Socratic thinking recommends a method for moral decision making in which decisions are to be determined not by emotions, but by logical examination of the question. One must think for oneself and not view the "commonly accepted" as the necessarily correct answer. Judgment is dependent upon critical and clear thinking. Action is dependent upon rational thought.

Teleological and Deontological Theories

Classical studies divide ethical thought into teleological theories and deontological theories (from the Greek words "telos" meaning "end" or "purpose" and "deon" meaning "obligatory"). Deontological theories are based on the premise that an action is morally right or wrong because of the intrinsic nature of the action to be good or bad. Teleological theories examine the consequence of an action to determine its goodness or badness.

One ethical principle is, "It is wrong to kill." Deontological reasoning proposes that it is wrong to kill because the action of taking a life is objectively bad. A universal obligation to act or to not take action based on the concepts of "divine law," "God's will," "natural law," or "conscience" are examples of deontological reasoning.

Teleological theories can be understood as one is obligated to attempt to attain a balance of good over bad. The balance suggests the presence of quantitative (or qualitative) variables and the ability to separate the whole into its fundamental elements. There is an implication of measurable difference between an action or judgment and the alternatives. "The ends justify the means" is the most common way of expressing teleological reasoning.

Would teleological reasoning agree with deontological thought in that it is wrong to kill? The teleological response would depend on the details of the situation and the desired end result.

Teleological analysis would examine the consequences of killing. A teleologist might argue that the killing of Adolph Hitler in 1933 would have prevented the loss of more than 10 million lives during World War II, and therefore would have been justified.

Graphic illustrations of ethical decision making can be observed in times of war. Traditionally, the majority position in most societies has been that it is right to fight for one's country. It is right to kill the enemy; therefore, it is a good act to kill. . .the good outweighs the bad. During the Vietnam War, many expressed the opinion that it was in this country's best interest to protest and not participate in active combat. Each viewpoint, fighting and protesting, presents examples of the same method of reasoning; by following teleological principles, it is possible to motivate contradictory actions. Conversely, many people—using deontological reasoning—refused to fight in Vietnam because they believed killing of any kind to be morally unjustified. For another example, one therapist might advocate treatment for a patient and a second therapist might believe treatment is not indicated. Both therapists proceed from the teleological principle that behavior should be in the best interest of the patient.

It is useful to subdivide teleological theory into the concepts of ethical egoism and utilitarianism. Ethical egoism promotes that one should do what will produce the greatest good for oneself. In contrast, utilitarianism promotes that one should do what will produce the greatest universal good for a specified group, such as producing the greatest good for one's country (Figure 4-1).

Moral Conflict

The study of ethics promotes critical analysis of issues or questions creating methods for the establishment of principles as the basis for decision making. Principles, generalized concept statements, ideals, or rules form the foundation from which judgments are made or action is taken.

But what if two or more ideals conflict with each other? Or, what is one to do if one feels morally obligated to take action and if one feels that the action will produce significant harm? The study of motivation, psychology, and human nature suggest other sources of ethical dissonance.

Moral conflict is the result of mismatched or inconsistent values. Moral conflict might be a consequence of a person's internal discord or it might reflect incompatibility between the individual's values and societal values (Figure 4-2).

Implementation of Morality in Society

Morality is an instrument of society that can become internalized by the individual. Social values codify behavioral norms for its group members. Certain kinds of actions are considered praiseworthy or blameworthy. Custom, ritual, and etiquette tend to remain relatively informal systems of social morality. Governing bodies have organized ethical principles into formal standards.

Law, statute, and ordinance are binding rules of conduct enacted by a governmental body. Regulation is instituted by associations or governmental departments, but generally

---

Figure 4-1
Reasoning Based on Different Ethical Theories

Deontological:
- Euthanasia is bad because life must be preserved.
- The fifth commandment says "Thou shalt not kill." Therefore, euthanasia which is the taking of life is wrong.

Teleological:
  Ethical Egoism:
- Euthanasia is bad because I want to be kept alive in case of medical advancements.
- Euthanasia is good because I don't want to live in pain.

  Utilitarian:
- Euthanasia is bad because generalizations could be made concerning what makes a life worth living (anyone born with a defect might be deemed not worth saving) but in certain circumstances euthanasia is good because it could curtail suffering.
- Euthanasia is good because it eliminates, in cases of catastrophic illness, the need to allocate expensive resources such as the cost of professional care, thereby stopping a financial drain on American families.

do not have the same power as statutes. Policy, formulated by agencies, associations, or governmental departments is considered less authoritative than regulations. Guideline is recognized to have less force than policies. For example, the Department of Mental Health can promulgate regulations, formulate policy, and issue guidelines and each would have a different level of influence.

Each governing body has the authority to formulate rules for its own membership. An obligation for member compliance to the standards and rules as a reflection of fundamental organizational principles is assumed by each governing body. Different types of governing bodies have been empowered to varying degrees but each has the right to institute negative sanctions when rules are violated. Thus, a municipal government has less direct influence than does a state legislature, but each has jurisdiction over its own constituency. Similarly, the American Occupational Therapy Association has regulatory power over its membership, while OT Licensure and Certification Boards influence and control activities of therapists at the state level.

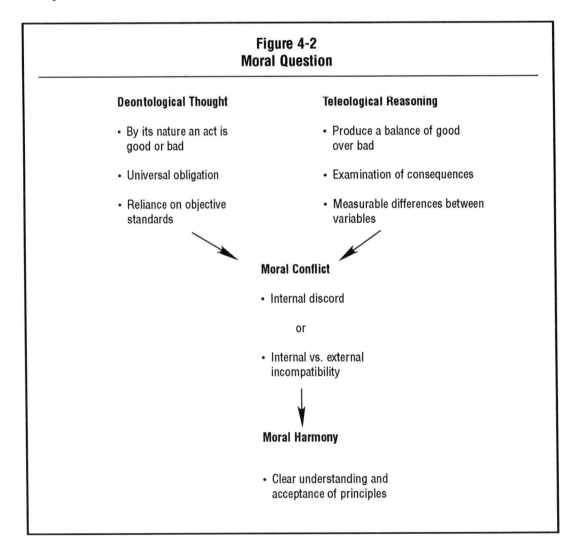

Figure 4-2
Moral Question

Deontological Thought

- By its nature an act is good or bad

- Universal obligation

- Reliance on objective standards

Teleological Reasoning

- Produce a balance of good over bad

- Examination of consequences

- Measurable differences between variables

Moral Conflict

- Internal discord

or

- Internal vs. external incompatibility

Moral Harmony

- Clear understanding and acceptance of principles

Principles of Occupational Therapy Ethics

As professionals, occupational therapists have an obligation to uphold the standards developed by the profession's governing body. *Principles of Occupational Therapy Ethics* was adopted by the American Occupational Therapy Association in April of 1977 and a revised version was adopted in April of 1979. Within the principles, it states, "As practitioners and educators, occupational therapists [must] keep abreast of relevant federal, state, local and agency regulations and American Occupational Therapy Association's Standards of Practice and education essentials concerning the conduct of their practice."[2]

The principles outline the values, the responsibilities, and the recommended and prohibited actions fundamental to the profession:

    I. Related to the Recipient of Service
       (clients, patients, students, and the employers of occupational therapists)
   II. Related to Competence
  III. Related to Records, Reports, Grades, and Recommendations
  IV. Related to Intra-Professional Colleagues
       (other occupational therapists)
    V. Related to Other Personnel
       (professionals other than occupational therapists)
  VI. Related to Employers and Payers
 VII. Related to Education
       (public relations)
VIII. Related to Evaluation and Research
  IX. Related to the Profession
       (to function as a representative of the profession)
    X. Related to Advertising
  XI. Related to Law & Regulations
       (to be aware of and function within the limits of applicable rules)
 XII. Related to Misconduct
XIII. Related to Bioethical Issues & Problems of Society
       (to seek information and determine implications for occupational therapy)

A revised *Occupational Therapy Code of Ethics* was adopted by the American Occupational Therapy Association's Representative Assembly in April 1988. (Figure 4-3.)

Figure 4-3
Occupational Therapy Code of Ethics[2]

The American Occupational Therapy Association and its component members are committed to furthering people's ability to function fully within their total environment. To this end the occupational therapist renders service to clients in all stages of health and illness, to institutions, to other professionals and colleagues, to students, and to the general public.

In furthering this commitment, the American Occupational Therapy Association has established the Occupational Therapy Code of Ethics. This Code is intended to be used as a guide to promoting and maintaining the highest standards of ethical behavior.

This Code of Ethics shall apply to all occupational therapy personnel. The term occupational therapy personnel shall include individuals who are registered occupational therapists, certified occupational therapy assistants, and occupational therapy students. The roles of practitioner, educator, manager, researcher, and consultant are assumed.

Principle 1 (Beneficence/Autonomy) Occupational therapy personnel shall demonstrate a concern for the welfare and dignity of the recipient of their services.
   A. The individual is responsible for providing services without regard to race, creed, national origin, sex, age, handicap, disease entity, social status, financial status or religious affiliation.
   B. The individual shall inform those people served of the nature and potential outcomes of treatment and shall respect the right of potential recipients of service to refuse treatment.
   C. The individual shall inform subjects involved in education or research activities of the potential outcome of those activities.
   D. The individual shall include those people served in the treatment planning process.
   E. The individual shall maintain goal-directed and objective relationships with all people served.
   F. The individual shall protect the confidential nature of information gained from educational, practice, and investigational activities unless sharing such information could be deemed necessary to protect the well-being of a third party.
   G. The individual shall take all reasonable precautions to avoid harm to the recipient of services or detriment to the recipient's property.
   H. The individual shall establish fees, based on cost analysis, that are commensurate with services rendered.

Principle 2 (Competence) Occupational therapy personnel shall actively maintain high standards of professional competence.
   A. The individual shall hold the appropriate credentials for providing service.
   B. The individual shall recognize the need for competence and shall participate in continuing professional development.
   C. The individual shall function within the parameters of his or her competence and the standards of the profession.
   D. The individual shall refer clients to other service providers or consult with other service providers when additional knowledge and expertise is required.

Principle 3 (Compliance with Laws and Regulations) Occupational therapy personnel shall comply with laws and Association policies guiding the profession of occupational therapy.
   A. The individual shall be acquainted with applicable local, state, federal, and institutional rules and Association policies and shall function accordingly.
   B. The individual shall inform employers, employees, and colleagues about those laws and policies that apply to the profession of occupational therapy.
   C. The individual shall require those whom they supervise to adhere to the Code of Ethics.
   D. The individual shall accurately record and report information.

Figure 4-3 (continued)

Principle 4 (Public Information) Occupational therapy personnel shall provide accurate information concerning occupational therapy services.
   A. The individual shall accurately represent his or her competence and training.
   B. The individual shall not use or participate in the use of any form of communication that contains a false, fraudulent, deceptive, or unfair statement or claim.

Principle 5 (Professional Relationships) Occupational therapy personnel shall function with discretion and integrity in relations with colleagues and other professionals, and shall be concerned with the quality of their services.
   A. The individual shall report illegal, incompetent, and/or unethical practice to the appropriate authority.
   B. The individual shall not disclose privileged information when participating in reviews of peers, programs, or systems.
   C. The individual who employs or supervises colleagues shall provide appropriate supervision, as defined in AOTA guidelines or state laws, regulations, and institutional policies.
   D. The individual shall recognize the contributions of colleagues when disseminating professional information.

Principle 6 (Professional Conduct) Occupational therapy personnel shall not engage in any form of conduct that constitutes a conflict of interest or that adversely reflects on the profession.

Note: As this book was going to press, AOTA was revising the Code of Ethics.

Reprinted with permission of AOTA, 1988.

Informed Consent and Related Principles

Principle 1.B of the *Occupational Therapy Code of Ethics*[3] focuses on one of the basic tenets of medical-ethics: informed consent.

Historically, the generally accepted standard of informed consent was a description of what was likely to happen to the patient based on the proposed plan of treatment. During the 1970s a new standard of informed consent developed. Medical professionals acknowledged the patient's right to be involved and participate in the decision-making process.

Informed consent is based on the principle that the patient must be given sufficient information for a reasonable person to be able to make a decision. The patient must be told the diagnosis, or if unknown, the diagnostic possibilities. The nature and purpose of the proposed treatment must be explained. The foreseeable consequences and the less likely risks must be discussed. Information must be given as to the seriousness of the risks and the degree and likelihood of danger. The patient should be made aware of the rate and probability of successful intervention. Treatment alternatives must be explained. The patient must be told about the likely outcomes if the recommended procedure is not followed.

Information must be presented in a manner that will reduce anxiety as much as possible in order to encourage understanding by the patient. The medical profession must include the patient as an active participant in the decision-making process. *Therapeutic-privilege* to withhold information is no longer accepted as a valid reason to avoid obtaining informed consent. However, *materiality* should be taken into consideration when obtaining informed consent. The notion of materiality infers that a medical professional needs to mention only the relevant issues.

Informed consent implies that the patient has a capacity for judgment or competence. Competency is a legal standard that examines ability to make a free individual choice. A person might be determined incompetent to give informed consent when of minor age or because of developmental, degenerative, or traumatic incident resulting in disrupted mental status.

Court rulings have decided that an incompetent person has the same rights as a competent person. The preferred procedure of implementing the preservation of the rights of an incompetent individual varies on a state-to-state basis. The right to grant or refuse consent for treatment can be reserved by the state court system or can be awarded to a guardian (family member or court-appointed) or a specially appointed team, such as a hospital ethics committee.

There is a recommended process useful in medical decision making for persons unable to actively participate in rational decision making. The concept of *best interest* is used as a method for decision making for incompetent individuals. It was described in a landmark case concerning a nonverbal mentally retarded 67-year-old male resident of a state school with an I.Q. of ten and mental age of two years and eight months who was in urgent need of medical treatment for leukemia.

> The significant decisions of life are more complex than statistical determinations. Individual choice is determined not by the vote of the majority but by the complexities of the singular situation viewed from the unique perspective of the person called on to make the decision. To presume that the incompetent person must always be subjected to what many rational and intelligent persons may decline is to downgrade the status of the incompetent person by placing a lesser value on his intrinsic human worth and vitality.[7]

There are many factors to consider when deciding what is in the best interest of an incompetent individual. The medical professional must consider if the individual had made wishes or beliefs known while still competent. Otherwise, the medical professional could make a determination utilizing the doctrine of *substituted judgment*. Substituted judgment involves looking at an issue from the perspective of the incompetent individual. Using substituted judgment the medical professional takes into account the current and potential awareness of the individual and examines the probable quality of life by factoring the anticipated benefits with the expected burdens.

For example, an occupational therapist assigned to Mrs. Jones, a patient with advanced dementia and hemiplegia, might contemplate, "If I was Mrs. Jones, what would I do if I realized that a splint could help functional position of my hand and prevent contractures? What if I also knew that the splint might cause pain during the fabrication process? Or while routinely wearing the splint, I might injure myself or have skin breakdown? And if I was Mrs. Jones, would it matter to me that the therapist's time spent fabricating and maintaining my splint might have been better spent with a different patient with a brighter prognosis?"

Quality Versus Quantity: A Moral Health Care Dilemma

The determination of whether treatment should be given or withheld should be based on the specific circumstances of the individual case, but founded on ethical principles. Just as the type of treatment should be based on well-thought-out scientific concepts, so should the allocation of treatment be based on well-thought-out ethical concepts. The basis for ethical decision making should be intellectual inquiry and not emotion.

Ethical problems focus on questions of what one is obligated to do in a given situation. Problem solving should include an inventory of the situation-specific factors. The medical professional should then follow by examining judgments made on comparable or similar cases, to determine all options and potential consequences of each choice, and decide on a course of action or, when appropriate, inaction (see Figure 4-4).

Traditional medical ethics emphasized a dual duty to promote good and to avoid harm. Serious questions as to the nature of "goodness" arise with increasing frequency because of social inability to come to a consensus concerning moral goodness. Technology is outpacing social policy because of rapid scientific advancements and societal changes. Enhanced awareness of health risks and better nutrition complemented by advanced health care

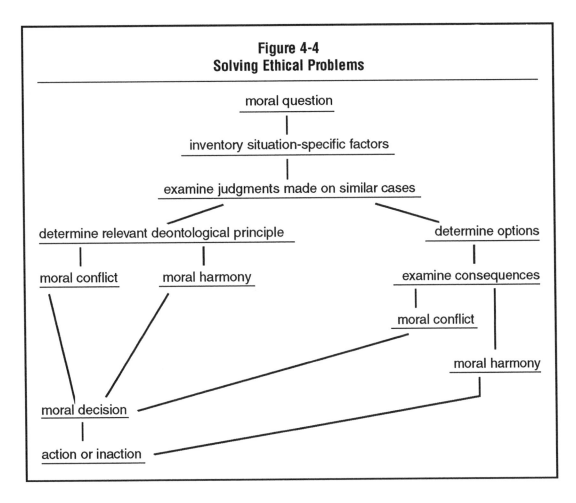

Figure 4-4
Solving Ethical Problems

intervention have contributed to a changing population. Demographic trends reflect a population living longer. However, there is a corresponding increase in the incidence of chronic or disabling conditions. A study revealed that about four out of five persons 65 or older report the presence of one or more health conditions.[4]

The importance for occupational therapists to be alert to social changes was emphasized by AOTA President Elnora Gilfoyle:

> We see rapid growth in health care expenditures, a consumer-driven health care market, increased federal legislation and regulations for health and human services, a rise in commercialism among health care agencies, industry providing wellness programs for employees, advanced technology influencing daily lifestyles—all accompanied by society's shifting allegiance from the biomedical model to paradigm of wellness with its concepts of health promotion, self-care, and productive living. We observe an expanding web of complex health and social issues, an alarming and critical shortage of qualified health care personnel, the graying of America, and an expansion of public education programs to include many functions associated with traditional health care services. We recognize the multiplication of professional specialties and subspecialties resulting in the resurgence of the multiskilled health practitioner concept.[6]

The health care system has become overburdened by increasing needs and increasing costs. The occupational therapist is faced with increasing demands and decreasing assets (especially manpower) resulting in ethical dilemmas related to resource allocation and distribution. Occupational therapists must give serious thought to allocation in terms of therapist time, and consequently, type and quality of intervention. The therapist is confronted with the question of whether one meets the basic needs of the many or gives emphasis to the few but most needy.

Payment issues add to the therapist's uncertainty. Third party reimbursement guidelines might conflict with therapy treatment goals by not allowing for coverage of preventative intervention or maintenance activities or in other ways limiting therapy. Must the therapist provide treatment without reimbursement or should the therapist seek payment directly from the patient? And what is the therapist's responsibility if the patient or the patient's family does not have the financial ability to arrange private payment? Is occupational therapy a service to be provided to only those persons who can afford to purchase it or is treatment in occupational therapy and health care in general a basic right?

When confronted with questions of this sort, the occupational therapist should return to the basic principles of the profession as embodied in the OT Code of Ethics, the responsibility and obligation of the occupational therapist is "furthering people's ability to function fully within their total environment. . .in all stages of health and illness. . ."[1]

Medical philosopher Paul Ramsey recommends a model of ethical decision-making. He begins:

> Our first move must be to agree on a term to express the ultimate requirement or standard or warrant binding in all cases upon the helping and healing professions. I suggest the word 'care' (or 'respect' for human life)—not 'care' in the sense of specific kinds of medical care, but 'care' as a strong, ethical expression, the source of particular moral obligations and our court of final appeal for deciding the features of actions and practices that make what we do right or wrong. 'Care' has the advantage of locating medical ethics within the ethics of a wider human community.[8]

Questions

1. Ethics is the branch of philosophy that is concerned with:
    a. Politics
    b. Morality
    c. Language
    d. All of the above

2. Ethical decision making should be based on:
    a. Logical examination of the issues
    b. Critical and clear thinking
    c. Rational thought rather than emotion
    d. All of the above

3. Deontological thought proposes that:
    a. One has an obligation to act or to avoid action because actions are good or bad by their nature
    b. One has an obligation to act or to avoid action by doing whatever will produce a balance of good over bad
    c. One has an obligation to act or to avoid action by following one's instincts
    d. All of the above

4. Teleological reasoning proposes that:
    a. One has an obligation to act or to avoid action because actions are good or bad by their nature
    b. One has an obligation to act or to avoid action by doing whatever will produce a balance of good over bad
    c. One has an obligation to act or to avoid action by following one's instincts
    d. All of the above

5. "Let your conscience be your guide" is an example of:
    a. Moral conflict
    b. Teleological reasoning
    c. Deontological thought
    d. All of the above

6. The purpose of the Occupational Therapy Code of Ethics is to provide all occupational therapists with a guide to maintaining high standards of ethical behavior. The code recommends that occupational therapists should:
    a. Take all reasonable precautions to avoid harm to the recipient of services
    b. Protect the confidential nature of information
    c. Be acquainted with applicable local, state, federal, and institutional rules and association policies
    d. All of the above

7. Informed consent is based on the principle that:
   a. Medical professionals should make treatment decisions based on scientific research and philosophical analysis
   b. Medical professionals should make treatment decisions based on the active involvement of the patient in the treatment planning process
   c. Medical professionals should make treatment decisions based on cost analysis and the availability of resources
   d. None of the above

8. An occupational therapist who works in an adult day health center has completed the fitting of a resting hand splint. Prior to splint fabrication, the occupational therapist took time to explain the purpose of the splint, the potential risks, and the probability of success. No guarantees were offered nor were threats made; however, the patient was told about the likely outcomes if the recommended procedure was not followed. The patient agreed to wear the splint. The occupational therapist used:
   a. Proper procedure for substituted judgment
   b. Proper procedure for obtaining informed consent
   c. Extraordinary measures beyond what is routinely required procedure
   d. None of the above

9. Best interest is founded on the principle that medical professionals should make treatment decisions for incompetent individuals based on:
   a. Cost analysis and availability of resources
   b. Social consensus
   c. Looking at the situation from the perspective of the incompetent individual
   d. None of the above

10. As a segment of the entire health care system, occupational therapy is confronted with critical moral issues that directly effect the type and quality of therapeutic intervention because of:
   a. Increasing demands for health care services
   b. A shortage of qualified occupational therapists and other health care personnel
   c. Lack of a social consensus concerning medical-ethical questions
   d. All of the above

Answers
1. b
2. d
3. a
4. b
5. c
6. d
7. b
8. b
9. c
10. d

Case Study 1

This was the second admission within a few months for Phyllis, a 72-year-old retired occupational therapist.

Medical history included radiation and chemotherapy for neck tumors and esophageal carcinoma. (Dysphagia and weight loss are common symptoms of this type of cancer. Possible side effects to the chemotherapy include lethargy and weakness.) Included in the history were recurrent depressive episodes, although last hospitalization for depression occurred years ago. (Symptoms of depression include changes in appetite and sleep patterns, low energy, fatigue, and a constant feeling of sadness.)

On admission, Phyllis presented with low energy, fatigue, and significant weight loss: symptoms that could indicate growth of new tumors, side effects to previous treatments, or major depression. Her primary physician made referrals including comprehensive evaluation (complete medical workup, psychological testing, and occupational therapy testing) followed by treatment as indicated by differential diagnosis.

At the next team meeting, the medical team was reluctant to make a firm diagnosis. Refusing to cooperate, Phyllis would not participate in standardized testing. Phyllis had gained a reputation as a "difficult patient." The floor nurses described her as uncooperative, demanding, and irritable. She complained about the food and refused to eat. She was too weak to ambulate. Mental status was alert and oriented.

Discussion among the team members focused on issues of competency. Was perception of reality impaired by depression thereby altering decision-making ability? Was Phyllis able to make rational judgments based on her actual situation? Did she have a right to refuse evaluation procedures that might disclose the presence of a life-threatening condition?

The psychiatrist proposed a course of electroconvulsive therapy, sometimes helpful for severely depressed patients without a clearly defined situational cause for depression and with a predominance of somatic features such as anorexia and insomnia. The team social worker interrupted the conversation by noting that if Phyllis was not transferred back to her nursing home by the next day, then she would be in jeopardy of losing her nursing home bed because of a Medicaid regulation allowing a maximum of ten days payment for reservation of a nursing home bed when the nursing home resident required acute hospitalization.

Following the meeting, the staff occupational therapist decided to visit Phyllis for an OT-to-OT conversation. Phyllis eloquently shared her thoughts about life. Having never married and without family, Phyllis made her work her life's focus. She felt the absence of her colleagues but, primarily, she missed the feeling of being useful and productive. She spoke about understanding "the importance of purposeful activity." Additionally, she believed that she experienced social deprivation. A speech impairment caused by residual damage to the vocal cords as a result of cancer treatment impeded conversation attempts. At her nursing home, social contacts were limited to two roommates both of whom had severe dementia. "Furthermore," she said, "my only remaining pleasure is no longer satisfying. Everything tastes funny ever since they gave me that radiation treatment. There's nothing left to enjoy." Phyllis clearly expressed a wish to be able to die in peace. Tearfully, she requested that the conversation be kept confidential.

The occupational therapist realized that she was caught in an ethical dilemma. By not explicitly disagreeing to the tearful request, was there an implied agreement to not share information? There existed an obligation to protect a personal confidence. Professional confidentiality issues were in conflict with professional obligations to provide a high standard of treatment and to avoid harm. What should the therapist do to best express her concern for the welfare and dignity of her patient?

Case Study 2

Mr. Jones was referred to outpatient OT, PT and Speech in a large suburban medical-surgical hospital. During an OT treatment session, Mr. Jones mentioned that he had received notification of paid costs for PT and Speech. OT was not listed on the insurance company statement. Mr. Jones expressed concern, "Will I be responsible for the cost of OT services? I'm on a fixed income and can't afford extra expenses!"

The occupational therapist knew that she had submitted charge slips to the billing office for the last three weeks. She assumed that a processing error occurred; however, the billing office assured her that the OT slips for Mr. Jones were received and appropriately processed.

At his next session, Mr. Jones brought in another insurance statement. Once again, PT and Speech were credited as paid but OT was not recorded. The occupational therapist described the situation to the director of OT. The director scheduled an appointment with the hospital fiscal manager.

The meeting with the fiscal manager was not going smoothly. He repeated, "We always do the billing in the same way. It's the only way to get reimbursed. If we don't get the insurers to pay, we get stuck with the costs!" The fiscal manager was referring to his longstanding practice of inaccurately billing third party reimbursement sources including Medicare, Medicaid, and the private insurers, such as Blue Cross/Blue Shield. He said to the OT director, "We always submit outpatient OT services as PT services. Not only that, but we always put recreation costs into the inpatient OT account; otherwise, the insurers deny us payment for recreation. We need every penny we can get because our overall hospital costs are skyrocketing. If the hospital revenue decreased, we would have to look at drastic cost-saving measures: maybe eliminated departments or reduced staff." The OT director responded, "I understand the problem and share your concerns. My loyalty to this hospital is unquestionable and I recognize the importance of fiscal stability. I am very aware of current economic and demographic trends in the changing health care environment. It is unlikely that Occupational Therapy will be a routinely covered service until third parties and consumers are made aware of the significant value of OT. Inaccurate billing practices are fraudulent. My department cannot receive proper recognition for the services that we are providing. Submitting costs under a more reimbursable label is misleading our patients, hospital administration and the insurers."

References

1. The American Occupational Therapy Association. Occupational Therapy Code of Ethics. *Occupational Therapy News.* pp. 24, August 1988.
2. The American Occupational Therapy Association. Principles of Occupational Therapy Ethics. *Am J Occup Ther.* 38(12):799-802, 1984.
3. Dyck AJ. Ethics and medicine. *Linacre Quarterly,* August:182-200, 1973.
4. Fowles D. The Changing Older Population. *Aging Magazine.* May-June:6-11, 1983.
5. Frankena WK. *Ethics,* Second edition, Englewood Cliffs, NJ: Prentice-Hall, Inc., 1973.
6. Gilfoyle EM. Nationally speaking: partnerships for the future. *Am J Occup Ther.* 42(8):485-488, 1988.
7. Liacos JJ. Superintendent of Belchertown State School and Another vs. Joseph Saikewicz, 373 Mass 728, 728-759, 1977.
8. Ramsey P. The Nature of Medical Ethics. In R Veatch, W Gaylin, C Morgan (eds): *The Teaching of Medical Ethics.* Hastings-on-Hudson, New York: Institute of Society, Ethics and the Life Sciences (Hastings Center) 14-28, 1971.
9. Welles C. Ethics and Related Professional Liability. In J Bair, M Gray (eds): *The Occupational Therapy Manager.* Rockville, MD: The American Occupational Therapy Association, Inc., 359-382, 1985.

Suggested Reading

1. Cassidy JC. Access to Health Care: A clinician's opinion about an ethical issue. *Am J Occup Ther.* 42(5):295-299, 1988.
2. Coffey MS. Brief or new—occupational therapy ethics self-assessment index. *Am J Occup Ther.* 42(5):321-323, 1988.
3. Fine SB, Bair J, Hoover SP, Acquaviva JD. Regulation and Standard Setting. In J Bair, M Gray (eds): *The Occupational Therapy Manager.* Rockville, MD: The American Occupational Therapy Association, Inc., 341-357, 1985.
4. Haddad AM. Teaching ethical analysis in occupational therapy. *Am J Occup Ther.* 42(5):300-303, 1988.
5. Hansen RA. Nationally speaking: ethics is the issue. *Am J Occup Ther.* 42(5):279-281, 1988.
6. Hansen RA, Kamp L, Reitz S. Two practitioners' analyses of occupational therapy practice dilemmas. *Am J Occup Ther.* 42(5):312-319, 1988.
7. Kyler-Hutchinson P. Ethical reasoning and informed consent in occupational therapy. *Am J Occup Ther.* 42(5):283-287, 1988.
8. Neuhaus BE. Ethical considerations in clinical reasoning: the impact of technology and cost containment. *Am J Occup Ther.* 42(5):288-294, 1988.
9. The Research Advisory Council of the American Occupational Therapy Foundation. Ethical considerations for research in occupational therapy. *Am J Occup Ther.* 42(2):129-130, 1988.

CHAPTER 5

Supervision

Bette Hoffman Harel, MS, OTR/L

Introduction

Supervision is an orderly process that focuses on enabling employees to grow and change. In developing supervisory skills, the therapist needs to gain a basic understanding of how the goals of supervision depend upon being aware of the adult learners' needs, applying various teaching strategies, setting realistic goals, utilizing basic learning principles and providing effective feedback. An understanding and application of these skills ensures a successful and supportive supervisory relationship. The supervisor who respects the capabilities of the learner and provides learning challenges matched to these capabilities engenders a commitment to the learning process.

In this chapter, the terms supervisee, learner, worker, employee, student, and staff therapist will be used interchangeably to refer to the person receiving supervision.

Definition of Supervisor

Supervision is an ongoing, dynamic, interactional process between supervisor and supervisee that enables the supervisee to grow professionally. The definition is derived from the Latin *super* "over" and *videre* "to watch, to see" (Webster's Collegiate Dictionary 4th ed., 1948). Consequently, a supervisor is defined as an overseer, one who watches over the work of another with responsibility for its quality. Much of the early and current writing on the subject of supervision comes from the social work literature. In the first social work text, *Supervision in Social Casework*, Robinson[15] offers a practical definition of "an educational process in which a person with a certain equipment of knowledge and skill takes responsibility for training a person with less equipment."

The Goal of Supervisor

The goal of supervision is to assist the supervisee in learning to perform the job in the best possible manner. The continued professional growth of the supervisee is measured by the increased effectiveness of the worker to apply clinical problem solving and occupational therapy skills and techniques in the day-to-day care of patients/clients. The American Occupational Therapy Association's Commission on Supervision[2] has broken down the goal of supervision into the following subgoals:

- To develop a sense of professional identity
- To increase theoretical knowledge
- To develop intellectual curiosity
- To solve problems in an organized and analytic fashion
- To make accurate decisions in a reasonable time period
- To be objective, flexible, and independent in thought and action
- To apply theory to practice
- To develop self-awareness and make changes in behavior on the basis of such awareness
- To cultivate individual abilities

To achieve these goals, the supervisory functions will need to be variable and complementary in nature. The emphasis on the differential roles of the supervisor will vary, dependent on the current and immediate need of the learner.

Functions of Supervision

The three functions of supervision can be divided into three distinct yet overlapping areas: educational, administrative, and supportive functions.

The education function is the most central responsibility of the supervisor with the goal of professional education and professional development of staff. The focus is on learning and performing. It might involve the direct transmission of information and knowledge, as in the orientation of a new affiliating student or a new staff therapist. Information includes orientation to the organization and department, including structure, function, policies, and procedures. Without this, there is no base from which to begin.

The supervisor teaches the learner how to explore a problem, how to understand it, and how to work on problem solving solutions in an orderly fashion. This provides the groundwork for moving the supervisee into independent thinking. The Socratic technique of teaching can be used, whereby the supervisor through asking questions stimulates thinking and helps the supervisee use knowledge in an appropriate manner. Another goal is to facilitate the learner to draw on what is known and to use knowledge toward the solution of another clinical problem.

The evaluation process has the primary purpose of teaching and is therefore considered a part of the educational function. The feedback, provided in the evaluation of a learner, directs the learner to focus learning on particular areas.

The supervisor, in carrying out administrative functions, ensures that statutory job requirements are met and professional standards, consistent with the profession and the department, are maintained. In this leadership role the supervisor sets the expectation that the worker will perform in a manner that facilitates the operation and management of the organization. The work of the therapist is overseen in order that the department's purpose can be carried out. The aim is to help the worker become self-disciplined in these matters. Other supervisory functions that are administrative in nature include delegating responsibility, planning, setting priorities, organizing activities, monitoring workloads, making decisions, and recognizing and solving problems before they are allowed to grow.

The administrative function places the supervisor in midposition. The supervisor is a person who has been given some official sanction to direct and guide the practice of others and, in doing so, is accountable to others. In this linking role between staff and management the supervisor must understand and interpret policies and procedures and how they work to support effective clinical practice. Because the supervisor is close to practice and observes the impact of administrative policies on clinical operations, it falls in the realm of the supervisor's responsibility to propose changes in policies and procedures when it is clear they impede rather than support clinical practice.

The administrative role of the supervisor is a vital and difficult one and might be the key to the effective flow of communication between varying levels in the organization. The participation of the supervisor in management processes will enhance the supervisors' ability to help assigned clinicians practice more effectively.

As in all new learning experiences, a degree of anxiety might be expected. New, difficult, and emotionally charged training situations can create significant internal tension in the learner. In the supportive role, the supervisor is required to note the learner's response as he or she copes with the pressure of new learning and the degree of stress in the process. It is suggested that the supervisor help reduce tensions by providing permission for the expression of feelings that help to reduce internal tension. By helping the supervisee identify behavior and feelings the individual can take a more objective and analytical approach to the situation.

Mosey[11] states the supervisee must be helped to accept the self, which can be accomplished by the acceptance of the supervisee by the supervisor, as a person and as a learner. Only realistic demands are made and the supervisee is assisted in perceiving criticism in relation to professional performance, and not related to the entire self.

On Becoming a Clinical Supervisor

Supervisors are not born from academic education nor from reading the literature on the topic. Many clinicians evolve into supervisory roles as a natural growth from clinical practice. It can begin by a challenge from a supervisor to develop supervisory skills by taking on a teaching function or supervising an affiliating student.

Occupational therapists who have performed well as clinicians, have an interest in teaching, and have been noted to enable others to use their capabilities start supervisory roles with a promising base. The knowledge and skills needed for supervision are basically the same as those that the supervisor possessed as a therapist, however, the method by which the knowledge and skills will be used will vary.

The developing supervisor will need to have at least a basic understanding of the administrative process because it will be necessary to interpret policies and procedures to supervisees in a meaningful way. Making decisions must be a process the supervisor can handle with a degree of comfort. Decisions are made against a background of understanding the department's practices. The supervisor serves as a ready resource to workers needing answers and provides guidance in helping workers in their attempt at finding answers. When the supervisor does not have answers, the supervisor needs to role model on how to go about finding the answer or determine an answer founded on a sound problem solving process.

The teaching role is a major one for the supervisor. The developing supervisor should enjoy teaching others and be able to individualize the instructional approaches to help a variety of workers perform to the best of their abilities.

Munson[12] has developed an assessment scale to assist would-be supervisors in rating their interest and readiness to undertake the role of clinical supervisors (Table 5-1).

Building a Working Relationship

Building Trust and Maintaining Integrity

The relationship between supervisor and supervisee is the medium through which a considerable portion of learning takes place and through which the goal of supervision is achieved. The process of interaction and communication is an extremely important one and can help or hinder the rate, quality, and integration of knowledge of the supervisee.

By using rapport building skills, the supervisor can be friendly and supportive, yet professional, convincing the worker that he or she possesses the abilities necessary to succeed. Expectations should not be set so high that the worker will become concerned and threatened about the ability to meet those challenges. By supporting ego strengths and making the process a positive one emotionally, learning is facilitated.

The supervisory situation must be such that there is ample freedom to communicate ideas and feelings. The supervisee's expression of both positive and negative feelings toward patients, the organization or other aspects of the work situation should, according to Mosey,[10] be encouraged in that it allows the learner to assess and evaluate perceptions. This process is an important bridge to increasing self-awareness, an important by-product of supervision.

Recognition of what is done well serves as a powerful motivator. Providing positive feedback about a therapist's increasing competence helps the worker accurately self-assess growth in attaining professional goals. The supervisor can meet valid dependency needs, and can expect there will be times when learners need substantially more guidance and assistance in learning a new evaluation or treatment technique or in problem solving a clinical or administrative problem. After addressing valid dependency needs, continue to challenge the worker to learn and work toward realistic performance expectations.

A Climate for Learning

The work climate can serve as a positive and supportive force for learning. The word *climate* is used to describe the network of messages constantly being communicated from our physical, human, and organizational environments and the interpretations we give to them. Learning can be facilitated or blocked by climate factors.[6]

Physically, supervisor sessions should be comfortable, affording some privacy and distance from distractions. This setting communicates a recognition of the importance of the worker and allows the supervisor to provide individual attention. The psychological climate should be a safe one where the worker can share weaknesses, struggles, and gaps in abilities related to clinical practice. No question should be perceived as too basic. Criticism can be expected to be constructive in nature, supportive, and based on reasonable expectations.

Out of this consistent base comes trust and a mutual sharing of questions, perceptions, and observations. It also contributes to a process of supervision in which the worker wants to be an active participant, rather than a passive recipient. With anxiety and threat

---

Table 5-1
Assessment Scale for Becoming a Clinical Supervisor

Factor (circle one for each factor)	Rating +	−
1. Enjoy teaching others	yes	no
2. Patient when others don't understand	yes	no
3. Skilled at indirect suggestion	yes	no
4. Commitment to helping others do better	yes	no
5. Willing to listen to others' complaints	yes	no
6. Enjoy planning ahead	yes	no
7. Willing to decrease my own practice activity	yes	no
8. Do not mind answering questions	yes	no
9. Do not mind asking questions	yes	no
10. Do not mind discussing organizational problems	yes	no
11. Can tolerate others making mistakes	yes	no
12. Can accept criticism	yes	no
13. Can accept failure of others to follow my advice	yes	no
14. Enjoy making decisions	yes	no
15. Do not mind discussing theory	yes	no
16. Need a lot of support for decisions I make	no	yes
17. Dislike evaluating others' practice	no	yes
18. Prefer to work alone	no	yes
19. Find paperwork a source of frustration	no	yes
20. Prefer action to speculation	no	yes
Total	+	−

From Munson, CE. *An Introduction to Clinical Social Work Supervision.* New York: Haworth Press, 1983.

minimized and growth, discovery, and risk emphasized, an environment is provided where positive and creative learning can occur.

Learning About the Learner

Designing any educational experience involves knowing who the learning audience is and at least a basic understanding of the level of knowledge the individual comes equipped with. Educational objectives are developed with the goal of "meeting" the learner at their current level and moving them along to higher levels. Learning about the learner is one of the initial tasks in the supervisory process. The supervisor must find out what knowledge and skills the worker brings to the tasks at hand. This process of evaluating the learner's current level of experience is commonly referred to in the literature as an *educational diagnosis*.

Such an evaluation might include learning about educational experience, areas of perceived academic strength, clinical settings previously worked in, familiar patient diagnosis, frames of reference practiced, preferred methods of learning, knowledge base, amount of supervision preferred, and goals the worker hopes to accomplish. This information can be gathered by direct questioning during initial supervisory sessions and supplemented by a review of records describing past performance from prior supervisors, reference letters, and autobiographical material submitted by the supervisee. Mosey[11] states that in addition to data about learners' skills, knowledge, and performance, important deductions can be made about the nature and degree of anxiety present, the current ability of the individual to deal with anxiety, present capacity to engage in creative learning, flexibility, and the ability to develop and sustain professional therapeutic relationships.

If teaching is to be effective, the subject matter to be learned and the student's way of learning must be related to one another.[3] Verifying where the learner is must precede where you want to help the learner to go. Taking the time to do a complete educational diagnosis of the learner helps to ensure this. This starts a continuing process and sets the pattern for the future.

Defining Expectations

Based upon findings about the learner's knowledge, skills, interests, motivation, and goals the supervisor should devise a learning or supervisory plan. This plan is influenced in part by the requirements of the job and the professional skills to be taught in the given setting. The plan is a working outline to be shared and negotiated with the supervisor. It might include a set of short-term expectations inclusive of the type and extent of patient load, responsibilities with regard to patient care, technical ability and integration of theoretical material expected, and teaching techniques to be utilized to accomplish objectives. The expectations defined should be considered subject to change. Alterations can be warranted for a variety of reasons: teaching methods might prove unsuccessful, short-term goals might be accomplished at a faster rate than expected, or a plan might include too many goals and therefore frustrate a learner unable to attend to multiple expectations. The collaboration of the supervisor and supervisee ensures that planning and clarification happen when developing, altering, or updating an educational plan. Coordinated effort and clearly stated objectives provide the supervisor and supervisee with consistent measurable expectations and definitive standards for evaluation of performance.

Basic Principles of Supervision

The Adult Learner

Training and educating adults is based on a set of principles that clearly differentiates it from the training and teaching of children. According to Knowles[10] the art and science of "helping adults learn" is termed *andragogy* and the "art and science of teaching children" is *pedagogy*. As the definition implies, there is more to adult teaching than imparting information, but rather a focus on helping and facilitating growth and learning. Knowles describes a set of assumptions about the mature learner:

- The learner perceives of him/herself as being self-directed
- A past reservoir of experience becomes an increasing resource for learning
- Readiness to learn is linked to developmental tasks
- Knowledge is sought for immediate application and learning is problem oriented

There are, therefore, a variety of implications for supervising the adult learner. Meaningful learning capitalizes on the more independent and reciprocal nature of adult learning. In appreciation of the self-directedness of adult learners the supervisor needs to preserve a learning climate that respects this characteristic of the learner. For example, providing supervisees with resources, a chance to access resources independently, supporting attempts at independent problem solving, and providing an environment where the learner feels accepted and respected are all supportive of the adult learner.

Supervisees come into new learning experiences with a storehouse of past experiences. Each set of life experiences is unique, and this accumulation of past experiences serves as a rich resource for current learning. Adult learning is primarily experiential and the preference is for teaching techniques that call for participation of the learner. Learners seek to learn that which is of current relevance to their particular stage in life. For instance, an occupational therapy student who is completing a senior college year and preparing to start a clinical affiliation in the area of physical dysfunction might have greater intrinsic motivation to attend to the clinical treatment techniques taught in class than to the "Budgeting for an Occupational Therapy Department" section of a course on administration.

Learning occurs during what educators call *teachable moments*. Therefore, a practical role playing session on transferring a patient with hemiplegia out of bed will be relevantly practiced on the job prior to the assignment of such a patient to the supervisee's caseload. The learner needs to learn and apply this skill now, therefore giving rise to the motivation to learn. The adult learner asks, "What do I need to know in order to solve the current problem that faces me?"

Basic Educational Principles

Each person learns at a unique pace and rate with strengths, weaknesses and previous experiences. The supervisor who has completed an educational and supervisory plan will better understand these differences. The following basic educational principles apply to the supervisory process and are the foundation upon which teaching-learning activities should be designed.

Principle #1. Meet the learner at his or her current level.

It is a good guide to start where the worker is and expect the learner to perform within current functional capacities. A show of confidence by the supervisor in assuming the ability to learn is a boost to the learner's ego strength. Beginning at this starting point ensures successful learning, provided learning experiences are designed to challenge the learner's current competency levels. It might be a mistake to assume that a student or staff therapist is competent in the therapeutic management of a burn patient/client after having recently completed a classroom review of clinical interventions. Understanding of actual clinical application might be lagging behind academic knowledge, given expected inexperience with clinical decision making.

Principle #2. Move from the familiar to similar but unfamiliar.

The ability of the worker to move from the familiar to similar but unfamiliar enables the supervisor to build on the skills the worker has. For instance, a new staff therapist who is competent in performing a range of motion (ROM) program with a patient/client who has Guillian-Barre has a foundation from which to begin similar treatment with a surgical patient whose status is one day post a total elbow replacement.

Principle #3. Involve the learner in the instruction.

The demonstration of a skill can have limited real or lasting value. The participation of the learner makes the learner more likely to own the learning. So it is important to ask, "How can I explain or demonstrate this skill or technique and how do I get this learner actively involved in learning it?" For example, a supervisor notes that a student fulfilling requirements to co-lead a series of therapeutic group activities during her psychiatric affiliation is not observing some of the dynamics between group members. The supervisor feels that since it is her first time co-leading this might explain the student's lack of observations. The supervisor can transmit some knowledge of group dynamics by providing the student with a chapter on group dynamics to read—but learning can be greatly enhanced by supplementing the reading assignment by designing an active learning experience for the student to document observations of group dynamics via a two-way mirror. After this active learning experience, have a discussion with the supervisor and student and co-lead a group again.

Principle #4. Proceed from the simple to the complex.

Arranging learning experiences by degree of difficulty allows the supervisor to provide the learner by assigning a patient/client who has had a mild stroke with primarily motor involvement before assigning a patient/client with profound motor, cognitive, and perceptual impairments. (Keep in mind, however, that easy tasks for some might be considered difficult for others.)

Principle #5. Utilize spaced learning intervals.

Design learning experience with intervals long enough to allow the learner to assimilate information but not too long as to interfere with application and carryover. A student who role plays sliding board transfers with the supervisor in the morning might feel equipped to attempt the transfer with a patient/client on that afternoon or the next day. If the student will not have the opportunity to apply the skill, the immediacy of learning can be weakened and carryover affected.

Principle #6. Facilitate generalization or transfer of learning.

Introducing patients with varied diagnosis to the supervisee should not necessitate returning to square one. The supervisor's job is to help the supervisee transfer knowledge from previously accumulated experiences to new ones. For example, knowledge of principles of hand splinting are applicable to a variety of clinical pictures; therefore, teaching the fabrication of all possible splint patterns would be teaching "splinter skills" rather than transfer of learning of splint design principles.

Matching Methods to Learner and Content

A teaching method or technique, in and of itself, cannot be considered valuable. As Austin (1952) reviews, "What appears to be a simple step—to impart knowledge—is conditioned by the variety of teaching and learning patterns that grow out of the personality characteristics and needs of teacher and student."[3] Learning activities must take into account the teacher's ability, the learning sought by the learner, and the job to be done. One of the essential skills in supervision, therefore, is the selection of a teaching approach and method based on information from the educational diagnosis or the prelearning assessment.

An organized learning plan that can be observed and measured is devised. These observable outcomes are often referred to as *competency outcomes*. The types of teaching strategies chosen will depend upon the nature and content of the material to be learned, the various needs of the individual and the comfort of the supervisor with the various teaching techniques. The range of teaching techniques will be reviewed later in this chapter.

Elements of Effective Supervision

A respect for and an understanding of the adult learner, combined with an ability to apply basic educational principles, provides a good base for effective supervision. Furthermore, effective supervision should, generally, be an enjoyable interaction that is structured, regular, consistent, and process oriented. The process aspect of supervision is as important as the content.

Research conducted by Munson with supervisees has revealed a number of factors the new supervisor must be aware of and prepared to deal with.[12] Although particularly relevant for beginning supervisors and supervisees, the beginning guidelines are applicable to many supervisory situations (Table 5-2).

Table 5-2
Elements of Good Supervision and Beginning Guidelines by Munson

1. The supervisee will likely have little experience at applying concepts and techniques.
2. Be prepared to demonstrate what you want the learner to do, at least initially, in new learning situations.
3. Periodically, the supervisor should observe the supervisee directly in clinical practice.
4. The supervisor should communicate expectations clearly and in sufficient detail.
5. Supervision should be based on what the learner needs in order to provide quality patient care.
6. The supervisor should be willing to share his or her knowledge and skills with the supervisee and should not be afraid, at times, to provide the learner with answers.
7. Adequate interaction between supervisee and supervisor is imperative.
8. Teach through actual patient examples rather than analogies or stories.
9. The supervisor, as a role model, should be committed to good practice and should teach through example.
10. The supervisor should check that the supervisee has enough work and sufficient challenge.
11. The supervisor should not judge the supervisee's performance in relation to other staff.
12. The supervisor should not criticize the learner's academic program, past experience, the profession, other professions or staff.
13. The supervisor should continue with own personal goals for continued professional growth.

Adapted from Munson's Elements of Good Supervision and Beginning Guidelines in *An Introduction to Clinical Social Work Supervision.* New York: Haworth Press, 1983.

The Supervisory Session

Purpose

The goal of the supervisory session is to improve the ability of the worker to serve the patient. It provides a forum for the supervisor to help increase the supervisee's knowledge and skills and the ability to apply these in patient care.

According to Abels, the supervisory session serves a number of purposes:

1. It is an opportunity for the worker to summarize and rethink recent experiences.
2. It permits a pulling together of learning.
3. It exposes the worker to others' thinking.
4. It gives experience in restructuring ideas and problem solving approaches.
5. It allows the supervisor to keep the worker abreast of what is happening within the organization and department.
6. It promotes team building.

Accessibility, Regularity, and Continuity

The supervisory meeting should be set at a regular time for a more formalized sharing. It should complement, not replace, the ongoing day-to-day problem solving mechanisms that occur in response to ongoing challenges. The new affiliating student will be expected to require frequent meetings with the supervisor. The new staff therapist will need fewer meetings designed to meet current needs. Assuming that all therapists, supervisors, and administrators continue to work toward professional growth with stated goals, the supervisory process, supported by regularly scheduled meetings, should continue with the goal of supporting that growth.

Plan on setting aside an individual time for each worker. At a minimum, a once weekly format is recommended. As for the question of how much time to set aside for each session, Peetes recommends the following as a guide: if the sessions continue in a productive manner and all agenda items are addressed, the time allotted likely is sufficient.[14] If agenda items are left over, more time is needed, or decrease the interval of time between each session. The supervisor is also responsible for knowing about the work of the supervisee and how it is being carried out. Therefore, the supervisor might need to determine how frequently a worker's progress needs to be reviewed to get this information. The same worker might need more or less supervision at different times dependent on personal and professional challenges that might face employees at different stages of their careers.

The issue of continuity is an important one. Sessions should have a flow just as treatment does. They should proceed in a fashion that allows for agenda items to be addressed in an orderly fashion, focusing on major points first. There should be continuity from session to session as well, with focus given to topics that require attention over time. If planned sessions are interrupted or canceled, reschedule the session.

From time to time content or process of the supervisory session can change but as Peetes points out, what is being recommended is not a model or format set in stone but "flexible supervision from a consistent base."[14]

Selecting an Agenda

Both the worker and the supervisor are required to think about the upcoming supervisory meeting. Learners are expected to take an active role, and expected to express needs, propose questions, and set priorities about concerns that challenge them in the role of learning therapists. The agenda chosen by the participants should be flexible in nature and might include:

- A priority order of the items to be discussed
- A summary of particular clinical activities the supervisor might need to know about
- A review of written evaluations, patient progress notes, and so on
- A continued exploration of an area of specific clinical relevance.

Developing a Supervisory Style

Munson states that style is simply the manner and patterns we use in attempting to communicate with others.[12] Style is also the consistent focus supervisors have in supervision, the manner in which their theoretical orientation is articulated, and the philosophy of practice and supervision and how they convey it to their supervisors.

The elements of style include voice, tone and volume, the use of expressions, examples, questions asked, and the organization and structure given to sessions. Style is as varied as the number of supervisors, and there is no right or wrong style. Supervisors, however, should develop an orientation or frame of reference to supervision that recognizes and incorporates their own personal style and strength. Remember that while developing personal styles and techniques for supervising, the primary responsibility is to the patient/client and the mission always remains to assist the supervisee in providing the best possible care to the patient/client. It is interesting to note that in a study done by Munson, most supervisors tended to supervise in reaction to the way they were supervised.

Supervisors should take the opportunity to be exposed to the work of other supervisors to help in developing their own style. In addition, feedback elicited from supervisees can help supervisors gain insight into their effectiveness. This is a valuable source of feedback and supervisors can see whether the learner's perceptions match the ones supervisors have of themselves.

Facilitating Problem Solving

Treatment planning is a cognitive problem solving task, which is the foundation of all occupational therapy practice. It is a fundamental process, yet one that is difficult for new clinicians to grasp. For a comprehensive review of this area refer to the suggested readings by Pellan, Pedretti, Rogers, and Trombly and Scott. The focus here will be on specific techniques to facilitate problem solving rather than a fully developed conceptual model.

As mentioned earlier, supervision should have continuity, just as occupational therapy treatment does. When a supervisee discusses treatment planning and problem solving regarding a particular patient/client, the case should be presented in a sequential manner. The supervisee should begin with the diagnosis, physical evaluation, cognitive perceptual profile, and functional status of the patient/client and progress to an assessment choice of a frame of reference, general intervention approach, and finally a description of specific treatment techniques and available alternatives. By helping the learner to study the patient/client problem in an orderly sequential way, the thought process eventually becomes an internalized mechanism for thinking through challenges in an effective and efficient manner. When problems are studies in isolation from the whole picture, you can lose perspective and the learning experience might be less valuable. Questioning is an important technique that supervisors can use to help learners reflect on their own work and learning. According to Munson, when and how a question is asked can be one of the most valuable forms of interaction used in supervision.[12] A simply stated question, which is clear and concise, can help a learner articulate knowledge and make treatment decisions. For example, in discussing the treatment plan of a newly admitted burn patient, the supervisor might present questions in a general nature to determine if the supervisee understands what treatment decisions need to be addressed. A general question might be: "What were the findings of the upper extremity (UE) range of motion evaluation?" If the supervisee does not present whether or not upper extremity splinting or positioning is required, questioning should be directed more specifically, i.e., "Do you feel UE splinting or positioning is required?" If either answer reveals lack of knowledge of what is needed, the focus of the supervision is shifted to the needed education.

Two levels of learning exist: technical competence and a comprehensive understanding of the total functioning of the patient/client. It is possible to have one level of learning without the other. It is important to promote both levels of learning although it might be appropriate to focus at times on only one level. According to traditional learning theory, technical obstacles must be removed before the higher level of perspective learning can occur. It is common to find that learners are more interested in technical competence and that it might prove hard for them to focus on skill development and processing at the same time. For example, a beginning therapist, intent on performing goniometric measurements on the dominant hand of a patient with arthritis, might not be able to relate the arc of motion available to expected hand function nor the impact on ability to manipulate feeding utensils. It is a good policy to focus on technical skill first and then progress to an understanding of the comprehensive picture.

According to Parham professional thinking involves being able to identify the reasons for the decisions and actions we make and that theory provides us with the necessary base for qualifying our choices.[13] She recommends theory as a useful tool for thinking and reflecting, and warns that an over-reliance on technical skills might ignore the broader context of a patient's/client's clinical problem.

It might, however, be hard at times for the supervisee to apply theory to practice. This is not unusual to observe, and Munson[12] suggests a guideline for helping learners by asking two questions:

- What should you do in this situation?
- Why should you do it?

The first question relates to technique, and the second is related to theory.

In summary, the clinical reasoning involves facilitating the supervisee to determine the patient's current status in a given occupational role, to describe what occupational therapy interventions can be done to enhance the performance of the patient and, finally, to make reasonable and ethical decisions about what ought to be done to enhance the functional competence of the patient. The techniques, used by the clinical supervisor, should assist the learner in attaining a model of clinical inquiry that is systematic and thorough. For further discussion, refer to Roger's Eleanor Clarke Slagle Lecture.[16]

Choosing Teaching Methods

At times, the supervisor can give the supervisee specific information or provide a reference source for obtaining the information. Reading lists, reference articles, and independent research into a topic should be matched with the current learning needs of the supervisee.

Discussion, case review, and questioning techniques, as described previously, help the learner arrive at conclusions in a logical manner. The process of arriving at a conclusion is stressed, rather than conclusion itself.

Demonstrations and the use of films and videotapes allow the learner to observe competent role models in the use of various professional skills. For example, the supervising therapist can demonstrate the proper method of performing a sensory evaluation on a patient with a hand injury prior to the supervisee performing a sensory evaluation. The advantage of a film is its obvious reproducibility. The learner can play back the information, attending to various components of the instruction as needed. The obvious advantage of the demonstration is the human interaction.

The use of role playing is a relatively safe way to give the learner experience with new skills without the performance anxiety, which might be present in the therapist-patient interaction. After the sensory evaluation demonstration, as described above, the supervisor might play the role of patient while the supervisee administers the examination. An even higher level challenge could be presented if the supervisee role plays having sensory impairment in the median nerve distribution to challenge the supervisee to analyze findings.

Problem solving discussions can also take place in a group setting. The supervisor can fulfill the role of resource person, encouraging group members to seek information and apply knowledge and problem solving skills.

As Munson points out "teaching may at times be more difficult than learning since a teacher must know how to let learn."[14] Being sensitive to the needs of the individual adult learner, incorporating some basic educational principles, and providing effective feedback do much to help the learning process along in positive ways.

Providing Effective Feedback

Feedback is the process for providing information about an event or behavior and in supervision it is the process by which learning and growth of the supervisee occurs. It is important to use feedback to facilitate positive change in the supervisory process and to do so in an ongoing and liberal fashion. The ultimate goal is to give information about a worker's performance in a manner that will enhance the worker's professional knowledge, skills, values, and attitude. It is the mechanism by which the learner hears the supervisor's assessment of performance, reflects on his or her own performance, and attempts change to more closely approximate the performance criterion for a given task.

In her article on *The Importance of Feedback in Clinical Supervision*, Freeman stresses "the importance of feedback is due to the fact that it can facilitate or hinder change. Feedback can help identify the next step in the change process, to clarify steps which have been taken previously, to evaluate whether a particular step meets performance criterion for a specific task, to evaluate whether it relates to or achieves the overall goals or other expectations as needed, and to identify possible barriers to goal achievement."[8]

Feedback can be constructive or destructive in nature. To be considered constructive, it should incorporate characteristics that will enable learners to accept and utilize feedback for its full worth. Following are several guidelines for supervisors that can be helpful for monitoring the quality and effectiveness of feedback provided to supervisees.

1. **Feedback Should Be Descriptive Rather Than Evaluative.**
   Feedback is limited to objective observations of what was said or done or how a task was accomplished. "Your initial interview with Mr. Carney wasn't done very well" is much different from "Questions regarding his family support system were left out." Feedback that is clear and specific is more apt to be understood.

2. **Feedback Should Be Specific Rather Than General.**
   To be told, "The standard format for administering the strength test was not followed," is not nearly as useful as hearing "You initially gave the patient the standard cue for the position to hold the dynamometer, however, the patient extended her elbow rather than tucking her elbow into her side at a 90 degree angle."

3. **Feedback Should Be Balanced.**
   The need to provide feedback should not be construed as something to be offered only when there is an area that the learner is required to improve upon. Feedback should recognize and emphasize strengths, provide powerful motivation, and nourish the learner's self-esteem. Feedback focused on the negative can discourage the learner and threaten his or her concept of competence. Although the scale might not balance for equal portions of positive and negative feedback, it is a rare time where tasks are so poorly executed that some positive performance cannot be found. The supervisor should make every attempt to avoid offering a positive comment, followed directly by a "but" and a negative comment, thereby neutralizing the effect of the positive feedback. For example "Your body mechanisms were safe when you transferred Mrs. Wood, but I felt you weren't clear to her regarding the sequence of steps." Instead, the supervisor might deliver the feedback separately to enable the learner to hear both pieces of information as distinct. "You need some more review in the sequence of steps for the stand pivot transfer. It looked like you were safe and secure in your body mechanisms with Mrs. Wood. I

feel with a little more practice you will be quite proficient in this transfer technique." The feedback is balanced and constructive and includes a vote of confidence for the expectation of improved performance.

4. **Feedback Should Be Well Timed.**

   In general, feedback can be best utilized when it is delivered immediately following or as soon as possible after the performance is observed. At this time the learner might be fresh in the reflection and review of performance and shaping of the learner's behavior might happen more readily. There are times, however, when giving constructive criticism at the earliest opportunity might not be indicated, and this decision should be made based on the supervisor's ability to provide well thought-out objective feedback and judgment about the recipient's readiness to hear it.

5. **Feedback Should Be Limited to the Amount of Information the Recipient Can Use.**

   The supervisor might feel compelled to offer the learner all of the feedback there is to offer, but information overload can prevent the recipient from utilizing any of the feedback provided. With too much information the learner is unable to set priorities in major areas in need of attention and might miss many important comments. More is not necessarily better.

6. **Feedback Should Focus on Behavior Rather Than on Personality.**

   An opinion that labels a learner with a categorical personality trait implies a static, fixed perception rather than a behavior a learner can change. An employee who is told he or she is "domineering" is at a disadvantage in comparison to the employee who hears "during the team meeting today you reported on your patients so completely that the other two disciplines did not have time to report."

For a complete review of characteristics of constructive feedback the reader is referred to Appendix 14-A in Casberque's chapter on the role of Faculty Development in Clinical Evaluation.[5]

Reinforcing and Building Skills

The reinforcement of learning is an important consideration in capturing and maximizing learning. Do not assume that one telling, showing, or practice session is enough for lasting learning to occur. Redoing or retelling or demonstrating again will ensure that knowledge has been integrated on a deeper level. The learner might not be able to request repetition or recognize its importance, so the supervisor should offer it and should do so in a nonjudgmental way. The second time a technique is demonstrated or reviewed the information is not so new, and the learner can attend to more dimensions, details of the technique, etc.

The supervisor might choose to repeat with variations for emphasis. After a therapist who has recently started a rotation in orthopedics successfully treats and discharges a patient with a total hip replacement, the supervisor can then assign a patient with a total hip replacement who has more complications that will need to be addressed in the occupational therapy treatment plan. This scenario provides the learner with reinforcement of prior skills and a new challenge as well.

Performance Appraisals

Purpose and Value

Assessment of worker performance is an objective appraisal of a worker over a specific period of time that reviews various aspects of the job. An evaluation should be a systematic judgment based on clearly specific, realistic, and achievable criteria reflecting the standards of the organization and the department to which the worker is responsible. By reviewing worker's performance relative to the job description both the supervisor and the supervisee learn the degree to which expectations for performance have been met and detect the areas where further assistance and supervision is warranted.

The performance appraisal occurs at the end of a predetermined time period when the process of learning and skill building is overviewed to determine if the therapist has acquired mastery or minimum competency levels. This formal evaluation differs from the ongoing informal assessments, which should be occurring as a part of each supervisory session. Both informal and formal assessments serve the purpose of monitoring developing competencies as the program of learning progresses. The formal performance appraisal is a time of stock-taking, concerning itself with the quality of performance and the quantity of accomplishments. The process can and should contribute to the continued growth of the employee.

The appraisal is a summation valuable to workers because it helps them know where they stand in the process of growth, obtain explicit approval for achievements, and gain a perspective in viewing change and accomplishments as a whole. Being systematic, this review can help the worker focus and better recognize and consolidate what has been learned as well as help to direct attention on knowledge, skills, and abilities that require improvement. Kadushin states "the evaluation helps identify the need for further goal-oriented teaching and is an assessment of present and past work, for the purpose of determining future teaching and learning activity."[9] It also provides a format for the learner to develop self-evaluation skills. Before standards for self-evaluation can be internalized they need to be defined in some explicit manner, as is done in the evaluation process.

The appraisal is of value to the supervisor and department as well. Administratively it serves as a solid base on which decisions are made regarding changes and increases in job responsibilities, including job promotions and pay increases. The appraisal assists the supervisor in determining if learning activities and teaching approaches require change and helps the supervisor plan inservice education. Above all, it identifies if the individual is fulfilling the goals of the department, which is ultimately to provide good therapeutic services to the patient. In this way, the appraisal is a process of indirect value to the patient as well.

The Productive Evaluation

Kadushin outlines a number of key elements for ensuring evaluations are productive in nature.[9] Each will be discussed briefly.

1. The informal evaluation is a continuous one, not an occasional event. The formal, periodic evaluation is a summary-recapitulation of previously reviewed assessments that have been done jointly in prior regular supervisory conferences. It should not contain critiques the worker is hearing for the first time and for which the worker is unprepared.

2. The evaluation procedures are discussed with the worker in advance and should include the standards being used, when it is to be scheduled, whom the information will be shared with, what use will be made of it, and orientation to the role of the worker in this process.

3. The evaluation should be presented in a way that communicates a sincere desire to help the learner to enhance professional skills and serve the patient in the best possible fashion.

4. It is a mutually shared process. Since adult learning is active learning, the worker should be an active participant, contributing to the evaluation. The worker can be asked to evaluate his/her own performance using the same form(s) as the supervisor. Each can prepare for the evaluation from their own perspectives, share observations and assessments, and resolve divergent views. This two-way communication decreases the learner's anxiety, allows a sharing of control, and respects the role and input of both parties.

5. The evaluation should be made with recognition given to the reality that factors can have impact on the worker's performance. For instance, the learner might have been faced with an especially heavy caseload of patients, unusually difficult patients, or a turnover in personnel that might have affected the day-to-day clinical operations.

6. The evaluation should focus on work performance and not on the worker as a person. This will be ensured if performance is reviewed in relationship to the specific duties assigned.

7. Strengths and weaknesses should be reviewed in a fair and balanced way. Look for recurrent patterns in performance rather than isolated atypical examples. Use legitimate, objective information to support observations of behavior and performance. Instead of using the term weaknesses, you might prefer "area for further or continued growth" or "areas for future growth" as alternatives.

8. The evaluation should be a summary that describes a process of accomplishment, an analysis of how things have bee done, rather than a good/bad system focusing on the points given to various accomplishments.

9. Use consistency in applying the same standards to learners with the same education, experience, and job description.

10. The supervisor should use this opportunity to be evaluated as well. The supervisee, likely, has very valuable feedback to provide and the supervisor who is not threatened and can provide a safe situation for the worker to deliver this feedback has much to profit.

11. Involve the staff in establishing the criterion used in the evaluations. More relevant criterion can be identified and it invites the commitment of the employees to the evaluation process.

Preparing for the Evaluation Conference

The supervisee can be helped to prepare for the evaluation conference by reviewing the evaluation outline and becoming refamiliarized with the job description. Self-evaluation notes can be prepared or the evaluation form completed with special attention given to accomplishments and areas where continued help or review is necessary. In a national survey by Kadushin a large number of supervisees reported that they were not given a formal statement that informed them of the evaluation criterion.[9] Only one in four supervisees were asked to formulate their own evaluation statement in preparation for the evaluation conference. Less than fifty percent indicated that they were given a written evaluation that was supplemented by a discussion. Forty-six percent reported that no formal, individualized evaluation conference was scheduled with them. When such conferences occurred they usually occurred at one-year intervals.

The supervisor is responsible for pulling together a representative sampling of the learner's performance for the time period being reviewed. There are many sources of information from which to pull. DeMers states that direct observation of performance is one of the most frequently used evaluation techniques in the health professions and is used in relation to several kinds of performance: knowledge, technical skill, interpersonal skills, and habits and attitudes. A variety of observational assessments, checklists, and rating scales are presented in DeMers reference on Observational Assessment of Performance.[7] Other sources are documentation of clinical evaluations and progress notes, a worker's verbal report of clinical activity, written treatment plans, reports volunteered by patients and patients' families, observations offered by qualified others, meaning other employees in supervisory positions who might have made observations of staff performance at team meetings, parent conferences, task group meetings, and in patient interaction. Observations by other professional such as physicians, charge nurses, and clinical specialists working with the therapist will help in providing a well rounded observational assessment.

Table 5-3
Performance Appraisal

BRIGHAM AND WOMEN'S HOSPITAL Exempt Performance Planning and Appraisal Form	Name	Title Staff Occupational Therapist
	Division	Department Rehabilitation Services
	Grade 702	Appraisal Date
	Supervisor's Name	Title

Section One: Key Responsibilities, Projects and Objectives: List key areas of responsibility, major job duties, special projects, and objectives for the appraisal period (about ten items). Sources of this information include the job description, institution and departmental goals and objectives, departmental planning meetings, and the like. The last item should be an "All Other" item.

1. Performs and documents complete evaluations upon referral from a physician; formulates appropriate treatment plans consistent with evaluation data.

2. Implements and modifies treatment program and discharge plans to maximize function and restore independence; evaluates, recommends, and obtains patient equipment and supplies.

3. Maintains and enhances professional knowledge and skills that include but are not limited to the fabrication of specialized orthotics and adapted equipment, application of modalities and therapeutic exercise, instruction in ADLs, and environmental design.

4. Professionally communicates and documents patient care; completes all other departmental duties according to departmental criteria.

5. Demonstrates effective interpersonal skills with patients and families; instructs them in individualized, independent therapeutic programs.

6. Participates in educational program planning, development, and implementation; provides educational experiences to department staff, students, and other hospital personnel.

7. Delegates to and monitors the work of assistants, aides, and students in performing physical therapy services.

8. Demonstrates time management skills and complete job responsibilities.

9. Performs other duties as assigned by rehabilitation manager or coordinator.

Table 5-3 (continued)

Section Two: Results Measures, Performance Standards and Importance Weights	Impor-tance Weight (IW)	Section Three: Results Achieved		Standard Achieved (SA)	(IW) × (SA)
		Description			
For each item in Section One, list expected results measures, and where possible, standards of performance that consider quality, quantity, financial results, productivity, relationship, and timeliness measures. Supervisory and managerial appraisals should include items pertaining to financial results expected, productivity, and overall quality.					
1a. Appraiser's judgment as to the appropriateness and accuracy of evaluation procedures selected and applied based upon observation and/or discussion with supervisor, and chart review	5				
1b. Appraiser's judgment as to the accuracy and thoroughness of documentation of evaluations based upon review and supervision of at least three patients' evaluations per rotation.	5				
1c. Appraiser's judgment as to appropriateness of goals and treatment plan, whether consistent with evaluation data, based on chart review, supervisory meetings, and feedback from other qualified evaluators.	5				
2. Appraiser's judgment as to thoroughness, effectiveness, and creativity of treatment program and discharge plans, modifications, and equipment recommendations based on observation, chart review, supervisory meetings, and feedback from other qualified evaluators.	10				
3a. Appraiser's judgment as to accuracy and rationale of professional skills applied; knowledge of trends and developments in the field demonstrated and integrated (based on observation of techniques, supervisory meetings, and feedback from other qualified evaluators).	10				
3b. Appraiser's judgment of the initiative taken to improve current level of skill and knowledge based upon review of education log and feedback from qualified others.	5				
4a. Appraiser's judgment as to thoroughness, completeness, and clarity of written documentation of patient's status and progress based on review of at least six charts per six month rotation.	10				
				Score:	

Table 5-3 (continued)

Section Two: Results Measures, Performances Standards and Importance Weights	IW	Section Three: Results Achieved		
		Description	SA	(IW) × (SA)
4b. Appraiser's judgment as to the quality and timeliness of verbal communication with supervisors, physicians, and other health care personnel based on supervisory meetings and feedback from other hospital personnel and qualified evaluators.	5			
4c. Appraiser's judgment of the thoroughness, accuracy, and timeliness of completion of daily tally and charge slips based upon review of at least twelve sheets and data submitted per year and feedback from qualified others.	5			
5. Appraiser's judgment as to quality, effectiveness, and thoroughness of rapport with and instructions to patients and families based on observation and feedback from patients, families, and other health care personnel.	5			
6. Appraiser's judgment as to the quality, quantity, thoroughness, and effectiveness of the incumbent's involvement in educational experiences and/or productive groups such as SIG, committees, task forces, etc. (Based on initiative taken, time to prepare and present, complexity of presentation or project, log sheets, creativity, routine vs. new and feedback from audience, group members and other qualified evaluators.)	10			
7. Appraiser's judgment as to appropriateness, effectiveness, and creativity of the delegation and monitoring of work based on observation and feedback from those supervised and other qualified evaluators.	5			
8a. Average number of productive units achieved during four random weeks per quarter. 6 = ≥24, 5 = 23, 4 = 21-22, 3 = 20, 2 = 18-19, 1 = ≤17.	5			
8b. Appraiser's judgment of quality and effectiveness of nonchargeable time based on observation and review of tallies.	5			
8c. Appraiser's judgment as to timeliness of completion of patient care responsibilities and nonpatient related tasks based on observation, chart review, supervisory meetings, and feedback from qualified others.	5			
9. Appraiser's judgment as to quality, quantity, and timeliness of completing all other delegated duties and assignments based on observation, supervisory meetings, and feedback.	5			

Source: Brigham and Women's Hospital Department of Rehabilitation Services

6 = Outstanding   5 = Excellent   4 = Commendable   3 = Meets Job Requirement   2 = Minimally Acceptable   1 = Unacceptable

Samplings of daily logs, tally sheets, and productivity reports can be reviewed to obtain information about time management skills. The supervisor should have access to much of this information because of keeping anecdotal notes of supervisory sessions in anticipation of the formal evaluation.

Evaluation Content

The evaluation should review all elements of the job description and it is useful to prepare an evaluation with specific, observable measures from each of the job description criterion. At the least, the evaluation should contain criteria that address professional relationships, knowledge skills and attitudes, observance of departmental policies and procedures, communication skills (verbal and written), initiative, ability to use supervision, and time management ability. (See Table 5-3 for performance appraisal example.)

Evaluation instruments constructed from job descriptions can be assigned numerical representation to describe performance levels.

The delineations in Table 5-4 can only be useful after each level is defined in as specific a way as possible. Scales can be developed that address abilities at above or below average; however, it is this author's experience that supervisees do not enjoy being associated with the connotation of average performance.

Mutual Goal Setting

The end of the evaluation should bring the focus to a natural closure of addressing future learning needs of the employee. Mutual planning for the future occurs based upon job requirements, performance expectations, and professional interests. Agreement might point

---

Table 5-4
Examples of Ratings and Descriptions for Standards Achieved

Example 1:

1. clearly above expected levels
2. above expected levels
3. at expected level
4. below expected level
5. clearly below expected level

Example 2:

1. outstanding
2. very good
3. good
4. poor
5. unsatisfactory

Example 3:

1. Consistently exceeds normal job requirements and is continually seeking opportunities for improvement.
2. Often exceeds normal job requirements and frequently seeks opportunities for improvement.
3. Meets expected job requirements and occasionally seeks opportunities for improvement.
4. Sometimes meets expected job requirements, rarely seeking opportunities for improvement.
5. Rarely meets expected job requirements and does not seek opportunities for improvement unless mandated by supervisor.

toward the need for more practice in evaluation skills, improvement in professional communication skills, experience with a broader range of patient diagnoses, or a need for more challenging job tasks, as in a promotion.

In mutual goal planning, the role of each party is outlined for the accomplishment of the stated goals. This completes a full cycle of learning about the employee's needs, setting goals, facilitating learning, reviewing goals, and reestablishing goals. Follow-up is mandatory as new goals are set. Follow-up is, most often, the missing component. Thorough follow-up can serve as an ongoing evaluation of the clinician, the therapy, and the supervision. Many errors of supervision are repeated because of failure to follow up.

Summary

The prior review of the dynamics of supervision points to the importance of the role of both the supervisor and supervisee in charting a course of learning, setting goals, achieving objectives, and reviewing accomplishments and challenges. The supervisor has various roles in fulfilling the job description, part of which is to help make the supervisory relationship a rewarding one for the supervisee. Worker satisfaction is linked to feelings of being worthwhile and doing useful work. Therefore, rewarding supervisory experiences will be those in which the worker feels he or she has learned, has been treated like an adult, and has been able to maintain integrity, even in the face of difficult challenges.

Awareness of the fact that supervisees observe and learn from the behavior of supervisors serves to remind supervisors of the importance of being a role model. Understanding the organization and department, principles of supervision and learners' levels, needs, and interests help supervisors to work with employees to develop organized learning plans with measurable objectives. A positive supervisory experience builds an atmosphere that encourages new ideas and changes and provides opportunities for each person to cultivate individual abilities. The learning environment should be set up in a way that enables people to do their best.

Questions

1. The supervisee is developing beginning competency in SOAP (S-Subjective, O-Objective, A-Assessment, P-Planning) note writing skills. Select an approach to teaching this skill based on the principle of active involvement of the learner.
    a. Provide examples of SOAP notes for a variety of patient diagnoses
    b. Review each SOAP note written and provide corrections for the learner to review
    c. Explain the different parts of a SOAP note and provide an outline to review
    d. After providing an explanation and reference, involve the learner in practicing SOAP note writing for a variety of treatment sessions

2. An undergraduate occupational therapy student is beginning a physical disability affiliation. She has no prior experience working with patients. As the student supervisor planning the first week of affiliation, which of the activities presented would you choose to include? Support your choice(s).
    a. Learn activity of daily living assessments and treatments for the patient with a total hip replacement
    b. Conduct a range of motion evaluation on a patient with an acute burn
    c. Complete chart reviews and initial interviews on assigned patients
    d. Instruct the family of a patient with a recent CVA in home management prior to the patient's discharge

3. The supervisor is providing feedback regarding the therapist's performance in a patient care assignment. Choose the best example of helpful feedback, regarding a long opponens splint made for a patient with a thumb injury.
    a. The splint appears to be designed well, but the patient does not appear comfortable in it
    b. You chose the right splint design, however the edges are not finished off properly
    c. You chose the correct splint design to protect the thumb. You performed the splint checkout thoroughly for most of the expected pressure point areas. The splint needed to be cut back at the distal palmar crease to permit full metacarpal-phalangeal joint flexion
    d. You molded the splint well, checked out the pressure point areas, but forgot to make a final adjustment

4. Which of the following represents the learning principle #2: Move from the familiar to similar not unfamiliar?
    a. Progress from instruction and practice of stand pivot transfers to sliding board transfers
    b. Progress from the fabrication of a stocking aid device to the fabrication of a dynamic flexion splint
    c. Progress from teaching a hoyer lift transfer to a maximal assist stand pivot transfer with a patient with balance problems
    d. In a psychiatric day treatment center progress from leading relaxation training group to leading a sensorimotor movement group

5. The supervisee is not meeting goals set in the time period allotted. Consider which of the following might be true:
    a. Insufficient supervisor time allotted
    b. The supervisory plan and methods may need to be altered
    c. All of the above may be true

6. Select a teaching sequence for teaching the skill of administering a standardized Perdue Pegboard coordination test.
    a. Demonstrate and allow practice time. Schedule a patient who requires objective coordination testing. Provide direct supervision as needed
    b. Provide a clinical training film followed by the assignment of a patient with dexterity problems
    c. Allow the learner to figure out on how to administer test in a standardized fashion
    d. Perform the test on the learner prior to having administered the test to a patient

7. The supervisor's main role is to educate workers. Therefore, the administrative task of discerning whether or not the employee is meeting job requirements and performance standards can be left to the discretion of the department head.
    a. True
    b. False

8. Finding out about a supervisee's past experiences, including job experience, patient exposure, educational background, and preferred method of learning is referred to as:
    a. Facilitation techniques
    b. Effective feedback
    c. A supervisory plan
    d. An educational diagnosis

9. The performance appraisal is not:
    a. A systematic review that provides information about future learning needs
    b. An evaluation that focuses on the personality characteristics of the learner
    c. A chance to reinforce and commend accomplishments
    d. An opportunity for mutual and reciprocal feedback

10. The supervisor's role is to:
    a. Help learners to think through clinical problems in a methodical manner
    b. To provide supervisees with the resources to find the answers to clinical questions
    c. Make sure that workers like the profession they have chosen
    d. Both a & b

Answers

1. d
2. c or d
3. c
4. d or a
5. d
6. a
7. b
8. d
9. b
10. d

Case Study 1

You are the clinical supervisor in the burn unit of an acute care hospital and Elaine, an occupational therapist with approximately six months of clinical experience, is going to be assigned to a three-month rotation on the burn unit under your supervision.

When you meet with Elaine before the rotation begins you describe the patient population, discuss the role of the various team members and role of the occupational therapist in the care of the burn patient. She is asked to come to this preliminary meeting prepared to discuss her prior experience on the previous orthopedic rotation, her perceptions of her clinical strengths and areas for growth, her goals for the upcoming rotation, and her learning style. To gather information about her clinical performance, you review the end of rotation evaluation prepared by her prior supervisor. These are some of the things you learn about Elaine as you gather the above information:

a. She is a better visual learner than auditory learner and has difficulty retaining what has been told to her.

b. After being instructed in what to do she appreciates the opportunity to practice on her own before the supervisor provides feedback regarding her performance.

c. Elaine feels a strength of hers is teaching the families of her patients how to carry through with exercise programs and activities of daily living skills.

d. Prior splinting experience is limited to the fabrication of two thumb splints for a patient with osteoarthritis of the carpometacarpal joints of both hands.

e. Elaine reports she is not yet comfortable in transferring patients who need moderate or more manual assistance, and is concerned about her safety in these maneuvers, given that she has recovered from a recent back injury.

f. She has a tendency to spend a lot of time speaking to her patients and providing social-emotional support, to the point where little time is spent on therapeutic activities. Short-term goals might, therefore, go unmet.

g. A primary goal of Elaine's is to be able to manage all aspects of a burn patient's care, including initial evaluation, positioning, splinting, range of motion exercises, activities of daily living, patient and family education, collaboration with other members of the team, reporting at daily rounds, and discharge planning.

Given this information, which of the following patients might you choose to assign as her first:

a. A 69-year-old male with a 50% total body surface third degree burn, affecting primarily his lower extremities. Social service expects there will be a problem with the discharge since he does not have a family who can help in his care when he is discharged.

b. A 50-year-old female with a history of alcohol abuse who sustained a burn injury while smoking in bed intoxicated. The burn affects primarily her face, neck, left upper extremity and upper chest. Her husband is involved in her care.

c. A 40-year-old female who sustained burns of both upper extremities while cooking on a camping trip with her husband.

Questions

1. Discuss the reasons for your choice of initial patient assignment.
2. Set competency outcomes for the splinting segment of a burn rotation. The goals should be objective and measurable.
3. Describe the instructional methods you will select and the steps you will take to teach the goals set in #2, given Elaine's learning needs.

Case Study 2

Consider the following scenario. The beginning staff therapist is conducting her first family instruction session. The patient is present and the therapist is showing the husband of the patient how to perform a moderate assist stand pivot transfer into the bathtub. The therapist has demonstrated prior to this that she understands the proper technique, however, the technique she demonstrates is somewhat difficult. The family is asking the therapist for clarification. You, as the supervisor, are looking on from a distance.

Questions

1. What will you do and what principles guide your choice of action?
2. Will you say anything and why or why not?
3. What will you say if you do choose to give feedback?

Answers to Case Study 1

1. c. This might be a good choice since this patient's care will initially focus on the strengths of the learner, i.e., teaching the patient's family to follow through with exercise programs and Activities of Daily Living (ADLs). The likely plan of care corresponds to the clinical skills sought by the learner.
2. a. Elaine will design and fabricate a well fitting custom resting hand splint performing a complete splint check-out and making alterations as necessary.
   b. Based on Range of Motion (ROM) findings, Elaine will be able to discern the need for an elbow extension splint to maintain and gain ROM.
3. a. Provide or direct Elaine to written and illustrated information on splinting given her visual learning style;
   b. Discuss how the patient's physical status may indicate the need for custom orthosis;
   c. Demonstrate the process for designing a custom elbow or resting hand splint;
   d. Involve the learner in the problem solving process;
   e. Provide Elaine with the opportunity to practice on her own before demonstrating her ability;
   f. Reinforce learning by repetition;
   g. Assign subsequent patient where decisions about splint needs, designs and fabrication can be generalized

Answers to Case Study 2

1. Initially it would be reasonable to allow the therapist to provide clarification to the family on her own; however, if there are safety concerns your immediate input would be necessary.

2. The transfer technique may be different but not necessarily incorrect. If the technique is incorrect, the therapist may self correct with the request for clarification from the family. This is a problem solving opportunity for the learner and your comments should be strained unless there is a safety issue or the therapist requests your assistance.

3. You will probably want to inquire about the transfer technique and have the therapist review the steps of the transfer. If the technique shown differs from what was taught, you may ask for the rationale for the change.

References

1. Abels P. *The New Practice of Supervision and Staff Development—A Synergistic Approach.* New York: Association Press, 1977.
2. American Occupational Therapy Association. Final Report on Commission of Supervision, Curriculum Study, 1965-1966.
3. Austin LN. Basic principles of supervision. *Social Casework* 33:411-419, 1952.
4. Brannon D. Adult learning principles and methods for enhancing the training role of supervisors. *The Clinical Supervisor* 3(2):27-41, 1985.
5. Casberque J. Role of faculty development in clinical education. In MK Morgan and DM Irby. *Evaluating Clinical Competence in Health Professions.* St. Louis: C.V. Mosby.
6. Clancy CA. The use of the andragogical approach in the educational function of supervision in social work. *The Clinical Supervisor* 33:75-86, 1985.
7. DeMers JL. Observational Assessment of Performance. In MK Morgan and DM Irby. *Evaluating Clinical Competence in Health Professions.* St. Louis: C.V. Mosby, 1978.
8. Freeman EM. The importance of feedback in clinical supervision: Implication for direct practice. In CE Munson. *The Clinical Supervisor* 3(1), Hawthorne Press, Inc. 1985.
9. Kadushin A. *Supervision in Social Work.* New York: Columbia University Press, 1976.
10. Knowles M. *The Adult Learner: A Neglected Species.* Houston: Gulf Publishing Co., 1973.
11. Mosey AC. *Occupational Therapy: Theory and Practice.* Medford: Pothier Brothers Printers Inc., 1968.
12. Munson CE. *An Introduction to Clinical Social Work Supervision.* New York: Haworth Press, 1983.
13. Parham D. Toward professionalism: The reflective therapist. *Am J Occup Ther.* 41:555-561, 1987.
14. Peters DE. *Staff and Student Supervision: A Task Centered Approach.* (National Institution for Social Work. Social Services Library; No. 34). London: George Allen and Unwin, 1979.
15. Robinson V. *Supervision in Social Casework.* Chapel Hill: University of North Carolina Press, 1936.
16. Rogers J. Eleanor Clarke Slagle: Lectureship—Clinical reasoning: The ethics, science and art. *Am J Occup Ther.* 9:601-616, 1983.

Suggested Readings

1. Austin MJ. *Supervisor Management for the Human Services.* Englewood Cliffs: Prentice-Hall, 1981.
2. Bergguist WH, Phillips SR. *A Handbook for Faculty Development.* Washington, DC: Dansville Press, 1975.
3. Dewey J. *Experience and Education.* New York: MacMillan, 1938.
4. Fine R. Some theoretical considerations basic to supervisory techniques. *Social Work* 1(1):67-71, 1956.
5. Haiman S. Directing. In J Bair and M Gray (eds.): *The Occupational Therapy Manager.* Baltimore: AOTA Inc., 1985.
6. Kadushin A. Games people play in supervision. *Social Work* July:23-62, 1968.
7. Mager R, Pipe P. *Analyzing Performance Problems or "You Really Oughta Wanna."* Belmont: Fearon Pitman, 1970.
8. Myers C. Some teaching method concepts. *Am J Occup Ther.* 17:187-189, 1963.
9. Myers C. Strategies in clinical education. *Am J Occup Ther.* 23:30-34, 1969.

10. Pedretti LW. *Occupational Therapy: Practice Skills for Physical Dysfunction*. Chapter 3. St. Louis: C.V. Mosby, 1981.
11. Pelland MJ. A conceptual model for the instruction and supervision of treatment planning. *Am J Occup Ther*. 41:351-359, 1987.
12. Rogers C, Masagatani G. Clinical reasoning of occupational therapists during the initial assessment of physical disabled patients. *Occup Ther J Res*. 2(4):195-219, 1982.
13. Trombly CA. Treatment Planning Process. Chapter 1 In CA Trombly and AD Scott. *Occupational Therapy for Physical Dysfunction*. 2nd Edition. Baltimore: Williams & Wilkins, 1983.

CHAPTER 6

Cost Management

Martha K. Logigian, MS, OTR/L

Introduction

Health care is one of the fastest growing industries in the United States, comprising 13.4% of the gross national product. Government spending on hospital care, specifically Medicare, has increased by 14% per year since 1966. In addition to inflation, 6 factors are cited for increasing health care costs:

1. technological advances in equipment and treatment procedures
2. greater utilization of ancillary services
3. increases in salaries and the number of employees
4. the advent of Medicare and other government sponsored health care programs
5. consumer insulation from the cost of health care due to insurance reimbursement
6. reimbursement for inpatient care based on the total cost of the patient's care regardless of the amount of services provided[4]

Because hospital charges and expenditures have risen at such a high rate they now face serious cash flow problems. Changes in reimbursement are unavoidable as hospitals are now under pressure by insurance companies and the government to conserve.[2]

Prospective Payment

In an effort to limit hospital spending, the federal government enacted a Social Security Amendment of 1983 directed at revising the economic incentives of the current Medicare program. Medicare, which accounts for approximately 40% of total hospital revenues, has transformed its retrospective cost based system into one of prospectively determined payment rates.[10]

Under this system, hospital discharges are classified into Diagnosis Related Groups (DRGs). DRGs were initially developed 20 years ago at Yale University to be used as a quality assurance tool for utilization review. The objective in designing DRGs was to define case types receiving similar amounts of hospital services. Length of stay was used as a measure of hospital services.

The current Medicare DRGs were formulated by grouping the diagnoses in the International Classification of Diseases (9th revision) or ICD-9 codes into 23 Major Diagnostic Categories (MDC). Each MDC represents a broad clinical category based on biological system involvement, diseases and disorders. Further division into subgroups lead to the formulation of categories of DRGs.

Assignment to a DRG is based on principle diagnosis, age, other existing diagnoses, principle procedure, discharge status and sex of the patient. The principle diagnosis is the one, after study, which necessitated the patient's admission. Each discharge has a specific cost or weighting factor reflecting average cost and relative resource consumption of the DRG. A hospital attempts to classify its case mix or relative proportion of various types of cases that they treat into their proper DRG.

The DRG based method pays a fixed amount for a period of hospitalization regardless of its duration or intensity of care. The reimbursement for a specific patient is determined by the average cost for the particular disorder or DRG and, except for unusual cases, is unaffected by the costs actually incurred in treating the patient. Special consideration is given to cases referred to as outliers and patients transferred between hospitals. Outliers are cases with either extremely long lengths of stay, labeled day outliers, or extraordinarily high costs labeled cost outliers. Day outlier claims are automatically reviewed by quality control mechanisms, necessitating good documentation by hospitals so cases will be approved. Cost outlier cutoffs take inflation into account and the updating of rates is accomplished by using the estimated annual rates of increase in the hospital market plus 1% to account for technological improvements.

Because an institution's reimbursement is based on prospective, fixed rates regardless of services provided, it is put at risk for costs exceeding the specific DRG rate and will have to absorb the loss. On the other hand, if the hospital treats a patient with a certain diagnosis for less than the designed allowance it can keep the difference. This aspect encourages the hospital to decrease length of stay. In addition, hospitals may be motivated to identify patients with less than average costs and avoid more expensive ones. Teaching hospitals and other referral institutions that tend to treat more severely ill patients may not be adequately reimbursed by a method based on the average patient.

This prospective payment system includes all Medicare inpatients but currently excludes psychiatric, rehabilitation and children's hospitals and distinct units within acute general hospital, long term care facilities, VA hospitals, and hospitals in U.S. territories.[3]

Controlling Costs

However, the Medicare DRG system is only a portion of the cost containment effort currently under way in health care. There are other cost containment strategies with which therapists must become familiar to successfully cope with the health care changes into the 21st century. Of the different strategies to control health care costs, alternative delivery systems such as ambulatory care centers and homecare are receiving a great deal of attention. Other strategies considered very important include: greater cost sharing with employees, self insurance programs, utilization review programs, second opinions, and pre-admission review.[4] It is interesting to note that the majority of surgical procedures requiring hospitalization no longer have preoperative hospital days allowed with the stay. For example, a total knee replacement candidate has all preoperative testing and teaching done on an outpatient basis and is admitted to the hospital for the surgery on the same day surgery is scheduled. In addition, the number of surgical procedures performed on inpatients has decreased, while the number of outpatient surgical procedures has continued to increase.

Costs can be controlled through shared services and group purchasing through the creation of multi-institutional arrangements, hospital chains, contract management, and corporate ownership. The "one stop shopping" concept is gaining support as a means to provide complete services in a community. A plan such as this allows the health care provider to address the whole spectrum of patient needs from the initial emergency room contact to home health care. This assists in early discharge, provides continuity of care, and reduces costs.[4]

Health Maintenance Organizations (HMOs) have grown significantly in recent years. HMOs manage health care to address critical issues such as efficiency, second opinions, cost containment through ideas such as contracting with a specific hospital for per diem discounts for HMO patients, or negotiating rates for per case reimbursement.

Preferred Provider Organizations (PPOs) represent the greatest growth area in terms of delivery changes. PPOs are an arrangement between payer and preferred provider that establishes prices typically lower than those established in the absence of a PPO. It also establishes provider utilization controls that include preadmission certification and length of stay review. With a PPO, a subscriber is not restricted to using only selected providers, however, benefits are more extensive when a preferred provider is chosen.[12]

Another cost containment strategy for health care is to establish a hotel or diagnostic unit within the hospital or adjacent to it. This is particularly useful for patients traveling from a long distance for surgery. They can rent a room in this unit and have easy access to the hospital for admission on the day of surgery. Typically in these units there is no nursing care available, only room and board. Cataract patients have found this concept helpful as cataract surgery is now done on a day surgery basis. Another example is to increase efficiency during a hospital admission through the use of managed health care plans. This refers to the concept of a patient care plan or protocol used by nurses, therapists, and physicians. It incorporates a planned hospitalization with expected length of stay and encourages consistency from person to person by clearly identifying the daily patient care to be provided.

Patients may require weekend treatment to achieve earlier discharge. Special equipment may be used to facilitate a speedy discharge, such as continuous passive motion (CPM) machines for patients following certain orthopedic surgery procedures. Discharge plans may be developed for the patient before admission. This helps to identify potential problems which may be encountered, such as long-term care requirements. It also allows the health care team time to resolve placement problems. By working as a team, length of stay is often decreased through these collaborative efforts.

Home exercise programs and family and community supports assist patients in returning home. Therapists need to develop a community resource file and get to know the people in the community to whom they can refer patients. This facilitates an efficient discharge and enables reliable referral to healthcare programs.

Incentives to decrease length of stay may include financial reward, space and resources within the institution. For example, as there is often competition over space, the reward for decreasing length of stay may be the long awaited staff lounge. Or staff may be sent to continuing education programs as a reward for cost containment efforts.

Finally, attention must be given to health prevention programs as a means of controlling health care costs. New prevention programs must be developed and offered to employees by providers and payors to health care. These include: corporate fitness programs, back schools, and occupational health programs. Programs need to address the needs of people of all ages, disabled or not, living in rural and urban areas. State and local authorities must increase expenditures for public health prevention programs and consumers need incentives to participate in prevention programs. The emphasis in health care in the future must be on technologies and interventions that enhance quality of life, improve access to care and preserve health.

Health Care Reform

During the 1980s, the key to a health care institution's success was increased patient revenue, often achieved through increasing patient volume. In the late 80s and early 90s critical shifts began to occur in the health care marketplace. Concerns over cost are a major issue, particularly for the two largest purchasers of health care, the government and private sector employers. This has led to an intense interest in evaluating the cost and effectiveness of health care interventions, as well as focusing attention on health care reform.

Thousands of hospital beds have closed nationwide as payors pressure patients to use hospitals offering lower prices. In addition, payors are looking for hospitals to shorten lengths of stay, reduce unnecessary utilization, emphasize outpatient versus more costly inpatient care, decrease expensive high-tech interventions, and offer price discounts. These cost-driven dynamics in the marketplace will be amplified by changes at the federal level once national health care reform becomes a reality. If fact, the recent federal deficit-reduction plan contains deep cuts in what the government will pay for Medicare or

Medicaid patient care.

In response to these pressures, health care institutions and providers will be forced to change the way they do business. Institutions are launching multi-year plans to position themselves in regional and national marketplaces. They are seeking to enhance preferred provider relationships in terms of both cost and quality. This includes immediate and long-term goals of cutting expenses, downsizing workforces, identifying program cuts and other opportunities to improve net revenue, including a reduction in the use of ancillary services.

Other efforts which promise to have great impact are interdisciplinary care improvement teams designed to streamline clinical procedures and services that are costly or use many resources, as well as examine patient satisfaction and outcome. Using Critical Pathways and other techniques, institutions are learning how to improve quality and cut costs for treatments. They are developing interventions that increase the efficiency and effectiveness of patient care. An example is the use of rehabilitative services in assessing the safety of sending patients home from the hospital and helping them become sufficiently independent to function at home.

These changes will present challenges and opportunities to occupational therapists working in health care. As occupational therapy managers, we must strive to understand the changes, and ensure that the profession is included as a covered service in the health care reform benefit package.

Budgeting

Adequate management information facilitates cost control by making available accurate and up to date cost and productivity data as well as information on revenue, charges, resource utilization and allocation. An effective documentation system (Chapter 3) contributes to data management. Computers (Chapter 2) are useful as they help manage data, from areas such as finance and materials management, and can be helpful in managing patient care data, budgets, equipment inventories, evaluation measures, and exercise programs.

Budgeting involves all staff, as 80% of the costs in a therapy area is devoted to staff salaries and benefits. A budget in a department of an institution focuses on two major areas: capital budget and operations budget.

A capital budget typically includes items and renovations which cost above a fixed amount, e.g., a purchase value or cost of $250 or more, and has a life of 2 years or more. These include buildings, major renovations and equipment such as a fluidotherapy unit. Capital budgeting is usually completed once a year. The process involves completing requests (Table 6-1) which are submitted to the administration for consideration for funding. Capital items are viewed separately by funding agencies with consideration for depreciation and possible tax credits, which is why separate budgeting for these items occurs.

An operations budget reflects day to day financial activity of an area. Commonly it includes timely information on volume, personnel expenses, non-personnel expenses and

---

Table 6-1
Capital Equipment Budget Request
Fiscal Year_____

I.   **Item**
      • Description
      • Vendor
      • Quantity
      • Unit cost
      • Shipping
      • Installation
      • Charge to cost center

II.   **Type**
      • Brand new item
      • Replacement item
      • More of existing item

III. **Justification** (What problem are you trying to solve?)
                    FTE, space, supply

IV.   **Impacts**
      • Financial
            (1) Expenses—one time
                    ongoing
            (2) Revenue—volume
                    charge
      • Others

V.   **Consequence of not having this**

VI.   **Rank order** (within your department)

---

revenue. It is prepared yearly usually 6-8 months prior to the beginning of the fiscal year. Table 6-2 is an example of a cost accounting report used to form an operational budget for each department in an acute care hospital. This type of report provides monthly statements of financial activity of the area/department. *Actual* refers to the amount spent, volume completed or revenue obtained for that month. The term *budget* is the amount budgeted for the month which is based on a yearly figure divided by 12 months. Monthly budget reports are provided to each area/department with detailed information on expenditures and revenue. These reports present the budgeted amount, actual costs and variance which is the difference between the two. Negative variance is demonstrated with brackets around the numbers while a positive variance has no brackets.

Volume is presented as the workload unit designated for the area. For OT, a common unit of measure is time or visits. To determine this a productivity system is useful. Productivity is a critical factor in controlling costs and meeting volume projections.[8,10] In

---

Table 6-2
Cost Accounting Report

Cost Center:

1. *Workload Unit*
   Units of treatment

2. *Total Personnel (FTEs)*
   Actual = all hours paid (productive and non-productive) as reflected in position control report
   Budget = total hours as reflected in staff plan

3. *Employee Benefit Expense*
   Allocated portion of benefits contribution made by the hospital as determined by an allocation statistic.

4. *Departmentally Budgeted Personnel Expense*
   Actual = Total Actual Weekly Salary and Wage
   Budget = Total Budgeted Weekly Salary and Wage

5. *Purchased Service Expense/Supply Expense*
   Actual expense for items/services used by the unit or individuals, e.g., phone, supplies, repairs

6. *Total Departmentally Budgeted Expense*
   Actual = Personnel Expense + Non-personnel Expense
   Budget = Budgeted Expense + Budgeted Non-personnel Expense

7. *Allocated Departmental Expense*
   Using an allocation statistic (e.g., % square feet occupied $\times$ \$___), a portion of the expense for each department directly related to the unit is calculated and expensed to that cost center

8. *Overhead Expense*
   Using an allocation statistic, a portion of the expense for cost determined to be overhead is expensed to the cost center

9. *Total Revenue*
   Treatment charges generated by the cost center

---

a therapy department, it involves establishing service requirements for the amount of direct care expected to be provided per therapist per day, i.e., frequency and intensity of services provided and the effect on resource utilization.[5] Questions that should be answered when productivity is considered include: Can therapy programs be done in groups? What equipment is absolutely essential for the patient? Should evening hours be established for outpatients and those patients admitted to the hospital late in the day? Are referrals prioritized and handled in an efficient manner? What is the appropriate number of direct and indirect patient/client contact hours for therapists?

To help determine staff productivity one method is that of a time based analysis, such as in Table 6-3. The information on this table represents data collected from patient charges. One unit is equal to 15 minutes of direct patient contact and a non-time based unit indicates the use of a modality. Charge slips which are batched and submitted daily to an institution's charge and audit department, list services provided for each patient treatment.

Table 6-3
Outpatient Rehabilitation Services Form

PROVIDER		DATE OF VISIT		
ICD9 CODE	REHAB DIAGNOSIS		**OUTPATIENT PT/OT 288**	

PHYSICAL THERAPY		# Units
Physical Therapy	0284	
Evaluation	0136	
Muscle Str. Eval.	0102	
Goniometry	0110	
ADL Function Eval.	0128	
Phys Capacity Eval.	1233	
Ther. Exercise Active	0169	
Ther. Exercise Passive	0177	
Ther. Ex. Coord.	0185	
Conditioning	0193	
Gait training	0201	
Prost./Orth. Tr.	0227	
Back Program	0243	

OCCUPATIONAL THERAPY		# Units
Occupational Therapy	1001	
Evaluation	1027	
Hand Eval./Mgt.	1035	
Percept Motor Eval.	1043	
Home Eval.	1050	
ADL Function Eval.	1019	
UE Physical Capac. Eval.	1217	
Therapeutic Act.	1068	
ADL Training	1076	
Coord Dxt. Tr.	1084	
Splint Fab/Adj.	1092	
Joint Prot. Tr.	1100	
Energy Cons. Tr.	1118	

MODALITIES

PHYSICAL THERAPY			OCCUPATIONAL THERAPY		
Whilrpool	0011		O.T. Modality	1126	
Hubbard Bath	0029		O.T. Intensive	1357	
Hot/Cold Modality	0045		O.T. Work Modality	1225	
Ultrasound	0052				
Electrical Stim.	0060				
Traction	0078				
Pool	0037				
P.T. Modality	0094				
Work Modality	1241				

EQUIPMENT

PHYSICAL THERAPY			OCCUPATIONAL THERAPY		
Ambulatory Aid I	0250		Adaptive Equip. I	1258	
Ambulatory Aid II	0268		Adaptive Equip. II	1266	
Exercise Equip.	0276		Therapeutic Equip.	1274	
Device Category I	1282		Splint Category I	1142	
Device Category II	1290		Splint Category II	1159	
Device Category III	1308		Splint Category III	1167	
Device Category IV	1316		Splint Category IV	1175	
Device Category V	1324		Splint Category V	1183	
Device Category VI	1332		Splint Category VI	1191	
Device Category VII	1340		Splint Category VII	1209	

This information is utilized for patient billing and development of a productivity report.

To identify an appropriate productivity measure, a regional survey provides information on comparable departments. Unique variables and constraints can be considered such as transportation delays, severity of patient/client illness and therapist's illness. A common unit of measurement is a 60% productivity rate or 20 units of treatment per day per staff therapist. Senior therapists rate is adjusted for supervisory and teaching responsibilities, for example a therapist responsible for ward rounds might only be expected to complete 16 units per day allowing 1 hour for rounds.

Each therapist (full time equivalent or FTE) is scheduled to work a 40 hour week Monday-Friday, unless assigned to work the weekend. For each day worked a therapist receives a 1/2 hour break and a 1/2 hour lunch. Thus, they are on-site for $8^{1}/_{2}$ hours, paid for 8 hours, and available $7^{1}/_{2}$ hours for assigned duties. Approximately 5 hours of a therapist's day is expected to be in direct patient care (chargeable) activities.

Included in the treatment unit charge is all direct patient care, note writing and chart review, portal to portal charge for home visits, and family conferences. Non-chargeable time includes: rounds, team conferences, set up time, professional consultation, meetings, teaching, student supervision, and educational activities.

An example of a productivity report is seen in Table 6-4. The report presents allocated staff, present staff and treatment units generated weekly for occupational therapy (OT) on the inpatient section of the department. Staff allocated (columns 3, 5 and 8) represent the number of full-time equivalent (FTEs) positions budgeted for OT/inpatient, which includes all productive and non-productive hours. The number of staff present (columns 6 and 9) represents only productive hours excluding supervisory overhead and non-productive hours (vacation, sick, holiday time). In this example, weekend productivity is considered separately. Most therapists find that they are able to attain a higher rate on weekends as interruptions and delays are minimal, as is non-chargeable time.

The personnel budget reflects all paid hours for staff including regular time, holiday time, weekend differential, overtime and benefit time scheduled and unscheduled. The latter can be referred to as non-productive time, i.e., vacation or sick time, professional/ conference time, etc. The statistic gives a true indication of the number of hours worked and the cost of each person in an area.

The non-personal budget addresses the supplies and expenses needed to run the department. For example, it can include office supplies, telephone, lab coats, beepers, travel and education expenses and splinting and adaptive equipment supplies. Other non-personnel considerations are employee benefit expenses, institutional overhead and allocated costs.

Revenue is the amount of fiscal reimbursement an institution can expect. It is usually based on the charges that the department generates. A cost accounting system which determines the true cost of treating an individual patient/client can be useful in determining revenue projections.[7,9] Such a system defines the units of service produced by each ancillary department, such as occupational therapy. It provides reports which enable department managers to monitor the variable cost of each unit of service over time and the full cost of ancillary services to determine whether the costs of patient care will exceed

Table 6-4
Monthly Productivity Report

MONTH: February
SECTION: Inpatient
THERAPISTS: OT

WEEKDAYS:

(1) WEEK BEGIN:	(2) WEEK END:	(3) # FTEs ALLOCATED PER DAY	(4) # DAYS IN WEEK	(5) # FTEs ALLOCATED PER WEEK (3 × 4)	(6) # STAFF PRESENT IN WEEK	(7) # TIME-BASED UNITS IN WEEK	(8) # UNITS PER FTE ALLOCATED (7/5)	(9) # UNITS PER STAFF PRESENT (7/6)
1	5	5	5	25	17.3	350	14.0	20.29
8	12	5	5	25	20.8	432	17.3	20.77
16	19	5	4	20	16.3	338	16.9	20.74
22	26	5	5	25	17.4	370	14.8	21.26
29	3/4	5	1	5	3.0	68	13.6	22.67

WEEKENDS:

(1) SAT	(2) SUN.	HOLIDAY:	(3) # FTEs ALLOCATED PER DAY	(4) # DAYS IN WEEK	(5) # FTEs ALLOCATED PER WEEK (3 × 4)	(6) # STAFF PRESENT IN WEEK	(7) # TIME-BASED UNITS IN WEEK	(8) # UNITS PER FTE ALLOCATED (7/5)	(9) # UNITS PER STAFF PRESENT (7/6)
6	7	15	1	2	2	2	45	22.50	22.50
13	14		1	3	3	3	72	24.00	24.00
20	21		1	2	2	2	43	21.50	21.50
27	28		1	2	2	2	41	20.50	20.50

Courtesy Department of Rehabilitation Services, Brigham and Women's Hospital

per-case reimbursement. Such a management reporting system is one based on Relative Value Units (RVU).[6] This system is both useful for management and practical to develop.

An RVU system is developed in five steps. The first step is to define outputs. An output is the service or type of therapy provided. Outputs are defined by identifying the variable costs for each service provided. Variable costs are those with no fixed value, i.e., the costs are changeable. To do this, revenue charge codes used by a department can be summarized into categories containing charge items with similar variable costs. For example, all occupational therapy fifteen-minute time charges are grouped into one category since they have the same variable cost. A therapist can provide range of motion, therapeutic exercise and homemaking activities during a one hour treatment session. The category would be called "Occupational Therapy—15 minutes" and the charge would be 4 units. Table 6-5 gives an example of output definitions.

The second step is to identify the unit cost standards for each output category. Because an Occupational Therapy Department budget consists primarily of salaries (80%), it is recommended that all department costs are treated as variable. Fixed costs are those which are not variable, i.e., the costs are not changeable. Equipment and overhead which are considered fixed costs can be captured in separate, indirect cost centers by the institution. Since output categories are defined as groups of charge items with similar costs, unit costs can be developed for each of the output categories. Expected labor and supplies costs are calculated for each category and added to find the total expected per unit variable cost for each category. For example, Table 6-6 displays examples of the results of these calculations for the output categories: Occupational Therapy, OT Modality, and a wrist splint. Similar estimated costs are developed for all output categories listed in Table 6-7, Column 2.

The third step is to calculate RVUs using the per unit variable cost estimates. The unit cost for "Occupational Therapy" (Table 6-7) is designated to equal 1.0 RVU. The unit costs of all other categories are divided by the unit cost for "Occupational Therapy" to arrive at the RVU value for each of the other output categories. The complete list of per unit RVUs is displayed in column 3 of Table 6-7.

Once RVUs are calculated for each output category, a common unit of measure is available for all different services provided by the department. This enables the fourth step of developing a management report to track unit costs over time. Ratios are constructed to find the actual variable cost per RVU for the department. These ratios are then compared with the budgeted, year-to-date, and previous months' variable costs per RVU.

An example of management reports can be seen in Tables 6-8, 6-9 and 6-10. The first report (Table 6-8) calculates the total RVUs for each charge code given the unit volume inputs. In this example, the volume of occupational therapy services are above budgeted levels for the current month (April, 1988). This resulted in the total RVUs being above budgeted level. This situation could develop due to an increase in the patient census and thus increase in demand for OT services.

Table 6-9 calculates the variable cost per RVU and compares the current month's figure with the budgeted figure. In this example, variable costs increased very slightly over budget, and the total RVUs are above budgeted levels. This caused the actual variable cost per RVU to fall below the budget level.

Table 6-5
Output Definitions

Occupational Therapy

Current Therapy Definitions

100	Muscle Strengthening	176	Jobst Pump
101	Goniometry	177	Fluidotherapy
102	Sensory Testing	201	Plastizote Collar
103	ADL Function	202	Neck Splint
104	OT Evaluation	203	Airplane Splint
105	Neuro/Development	204	Humeral Fracture Splint
106	Hand Evaluation	205	Elbow Splint
107	Prosthetic/Orthotic Education	206	Elbow Hinge Splint
108	Perceptual Motor	207	Wrist Splint
109	Cognitive Evaluation	208	Wrist Hinge Splint
110	Home Evaluation	209	Finger/Wrist Splint
111	Vocational Evaluation	210	Thumb/Wrist Splint
150	Therapeutic Exercise	211	Hand Resting Splint
152	Sensory Re-Education	212	Burn Hand Splint
153	Perceptual Motor Training	213	Dynamic Flexion Splint
154	ADL Training	214	Dynamic Extension Splint
155	Coordination Dexterity Training	215	Bunnell Splint
156	Dysphagia Training	216	Finger Gutter Splint
157	Splint Fabrication	217	Aluminum Finger Splint
158	Joint Protection Training	218	CMC Splint
159	Energy Conservation Training	219	Knee Cylinder Splint
160	Patient/Family Education	220	Hallox Valgus Splint
161	Prosthetic Training	221	Foot/Ankle Large Splint
165	Telemetry		

Table 6-5 (continued)
Output Definitions

1. Occupational Therapy—15 minutes
   (add current 100-161)

2. Occupational Therapy Modality
   (add current 175-177)

3. Splint Category 1
   (add current 215-218, 220)

4. Splint Category 2
   (add current 207-210, 213, 214)

5. Splint Category 3
   (add current 201, 211, 212)

6. Splint Category 4
   (add current 202, 204, 205)

7. Splint Category 5
   (add current 206)

8. Splint Category 5
   (add current 219)

9. Splint Category 7
   (add current 203, 221)

Table 6-10 provides a trend analysis of unit costs. Actual cost per RVU figures for each month are compared with the budgeted and year-to-date average levels. In this example, it is found that unit costs are above the budgeted level in February and March dropped below budgeted level in April.

The fifth step is the development of transfer prices which represent the total (variable plus fixed) cost of each type of service. Total costs are needed as they are used to calculate the cost-per-case for analysis of DRGs. As variable costs have been calculated for each charge code, fixed costs must be determined. To find fixed costs, cost reports and cost allocation statistics are studied to estimate the fraction of hospital-wide indirect overhead costs which should be assigned to an Occupational Therapy department, using a refined step-down methodology.[11] Once total fixed costs are identified, this figure is divided by the budgeted total RVUs to find the budgeted fixed cost per RVU (Column 4, Table 6-11). The fixed cost of each type of therapy was found by multiplying the budgeted indirect cost per RVU by the total RVUs assigned to each charge code. The variable and fixed costs are then added for each charge code to find the total cost used as the transfer price (Column 5, Table 6-11).

The figures in Table 6-11 range from $5.90 to $251.37, but the absolute dollar amount is not important. Occupational therapy at $5.70 is provided to patients much more often than a splint in category 7 at $251.37. The important point is that the costs transferred to the cost-per-case analyses represent all hospital-related costs of providing occupational therapy to patients.

One recurring issue in designing cost accounting systems is distinguishing fixed from variable costs. This system is a straightforward breakdown: labor and supplies are deemed variable and equipment and overhead are deemed fixed. In some cases, this type of

Table 6-6
Identifying Variable Costs For Each Output Category

Charge Code/Output	(1) Time	(2) Average Wage (Salary + 24% fringe)	(3) Total Time Cost (1 × 2)	(4) Materials Costs	(5) Total Variable Cost (3 + 4)
Occupational Therapy	15 min	$0.25/min	$3.60	$0.00	$3.60
OT Modality	60 min	$0.24/min	$14.20	$6.32	$20.52
Splint Category 2 (*wrist splint)	0 min	$0.24/min	$0.00	$19.80	$19.80

*Splint Fabrication time is included in "Occupational Therapy" time unit charge.

Calculating Variable Cost of Each Charge Code

Splint	(1) Splinting Material	(2) Splinting Material Cost	(3) Velcro Cost	(4) Total Material Cost (2 + 3)
Wrist Splint	Orthoplast	$17.00	$2.80	$19.80

Table 6-7
Calculating Relative Value Units (RVUs) Using Variable Costs
(1)	(2)	(3)
Charges Codes: Treatment	Variable Cost per Charge Code	RVUs per Charge Code (2)-3.60
101: Occupational Therapy (15 min)	$ 3.60	1.0
102: OT Modality	$ 20.52	5.7
103: Splint Category 1	$ 6.48	1.8
104: Splint Category 2	$ 19.80	5.5
105: Splint Category 3	$ 33.12	9.2
106: Splint Category 4	$ 46.44	12.9
107: Splint Category 5	$ 59.40	16.5
108: Splint Category 6	$ 99.36	27.6
109: Splint Category 7	$158.76	44.1

Table 6-8
Relative Value Unit (RVU) Report For April, 1988, Department of Rehabilitation Services
(Cost Center: Inpatient Occupational Therapy)

Cost Center Output Categories	(1) Actual April, 1988 Unit Volume	(2) Budgeted Monthly Unit Volume	(3) Per Unit RVUs	(4) Total Actual RVUs (1 × 3)	(5) Budgeted RVUs (2 × 3)
Occupational Therapy	1,575	1,500	1.0	1,575.0	1,500.0
OT Modality	7	5	5.7	39.9	28.5
Splint Category 1	2	1	1.8	3.6	1.8
Splint Category 2	3	2	5.5	16.5	11.0
Splint Category 3	4	0	9.2	36.8	0.0
Splint Category 4	3	3	12.9	38.7	38.7
Splint Category 5	2	0	16.5	33.0	0.0
Splint Category 6	2	1	27.6	55.2	27.6
Splint Category 7	2	0	44.1	88.2	0.0
Cost Center Total RVUs				1,886.9	1,607.6

Note: OT = Occupational Therapy

Table 6-9
Variable Cost Per Relative Value Unit (RVU) Report: Flexible Budget Analysis For April, 1988
(Cost Center: Inpatient Therapy)

(1) Total RVUs	(2) Variable Costs*	(3) Variable Cost per RVU (2/1)	(4) Budgeted RVUs	(5) Budgeted Variable Costs	(6) Budgeted Variable Costs per RVU (5/4)
1,887	$5,799	$3.07	1,608	$5,790	$3.60

*Variable costs are determined from monthly department budget reports which indicate salaries and expenses for the month

Table 6-10
Trend Report: Variable Cost Per Relative Value Unit (RVU)
(Cost Center: Inpatient Occupational Therapy)

(1) Budgeted	(2) YTDA	(3) February	(4) March	(5) April	(6) May
$3.60	$3.47	$3.65	$3.70	$3.07	

YTDA = year to date average

Table 6-11
Transfer Prices for Rehabilitation Services

(1)	(2)	(3)	(4)	(5)
Output Categories	Per Unit RVUs	Variable Cost (2) x $3.60*	Fixed Cost (2) x $2.10**	Transfer Price (3) + (4)
1. Occupational Therapy	1.0	$ 3.60	$ 2.10	$ 5.70
2. OT Modality	5.7	$ 20.52	$11.97	$ 32.49
3. Splint Category 1	1.8	$ 6.48	$ 3.78	$ 10.26
4. Splint Category 2	5.5	$ 19.80	$11.55	$ 31.35
5. Splint Category 3	9.2	$ 33.12	$19.32	$ 52.44
6. Splint Category 4	12.9	$ 46.44	$27.09	$ 73.53
7. Splint Category 5	16.5	$ 59.40	$34.65	$ 94.05
8. Splint Category 6	27.6	$ 99.36	$57.96	$157.32
9. Splint Category 7	44.1	$158.76	$92.61	$251.37

Budgeted Variable Cost per RVU = $3.60
**Budgeted Fixed Cost per RVU = $2.1*

breakdown may seem to create a distortion. Certain types of personnel costs, e.g., supervisors and managers are usually viewed as semi-fixed costs. But this system encourages managers to critically evaluate the breakdown of their time to encourage them to see more patients. If they see more patients while staff therapists maintain their patient care service levels, the unit cost of care will decrease.

Also, the system is not intended to highlight month-to-month fluctuations in unit costs, which could be affected by changing patient loads spread over inflexible semi-fixed costs. Rather, it highlights trends in unit costs over three or four month periods, when unit costs should be controllable even given fluctuations in patient census. This longer-term view is intended to encourage cost reduction by attrition instead of layoffs by providing managers several months to adjust to decreasing patient volume.

Management reporting systems implemented in all ancillary departments should be linked to a cost-per-case management system to be most effective in reducing costs. Only

---

Table 6-12
Outpatient Upper Extremity Management Program

This cost analysis was prepared for a proposed merge of outpatient occupational therapy with
a new outpatient upper extremity program.

Personnel	FTE	Cost
Orthopedic Surgeon (Hand Specialist)	0.20	$25,875
Neurologist	0.10	12,938
Hand Fellow	0.25	8,840
Occupational Therapist	1.00	43,680
Physical Therapist	0.50	19,760
Receptionist	0.50	12,843
Hand Therapist	0.50	18,000
Fringe (24%)		33,598
Total		**$175,534**
Non-personnel Expenses not Previously Budgeted		
Space 1400 square feet ($29/sq ft)		$40,600
Phone - New		1,143
Supplies - New		3,500
Other Direct Expenses (Based on 2/3 FY 1990 OPD-OT)		14,711
Total Direct Non-personnel		**$59,954**
Allocated and Overhead (Based on 1/2 FY 1990 OPD-OT Major Allocation Related to Space)		$98,093
Extra Depreciation - New Equipment for Upper Extremity Program		4,100
Total Other Expenses		**$102,193**

with an integrated system are assigned costs under the control of the individuals held accountable for these costs. Physicians are responsible for the cost implications of the patients' length of stay and frequency of therapies and tests while ancillary department managers are responsible for the unit cost of providing those services.

Table 6-12 presents a cost analysis for an upper extremity management program. It lists the components mentioned in this chapter. An analysis reveals that this proposal should clear $133,071 in gross revenue, which suggests that this should be a successful program.

Questions

1. To justify the need for more OT aides in a large OT department, you would:
    a. Need to determine current staff productivity.
    b. Establish service requirements for all staff.
    c. None of the above.
    d. a and b.

2. Which of the following help to decrease length of stay in an acute care hospital?
    a. Establishing a hotel or diagnostic unit adjacent the hospital.
    b. Providing pre-admission testing and outpatient teaching.
    c. Providing weekend occupational therapy.
    d. All of the above.

3. Hospital costs have increased because of:
    a. Greater utilization of ancillary services.
    b. An increase in government sponsored health care programs.
    c. Salary increases for health care workers.
    d. All of the above.

4. DRG stands for:
    a. Disability Related Groups.
    b. Diagnosis Related Groups.
    c. Diagnosis Regulated Government Intervention.
    d. None of the above.

5. Ways for hospitals to control costs include:
    a. Decreasing length of stay.
    b. Increasing productivity.
    c. Implementing managed health care plans.
    d. All of the above.

6. To define outputs, the OT Department must:
    a. Summarize into categories charge items with similar variable cost.
    b. Only summarize fixed costs.
    c. a and b.
    d. None of the above.

7. Which of the following statements are true:
    a. Management reporting systems should be linked to cost-per-case analysis.
    b. Productivity should not be linked to cost control strategies.
    c. Physicians are the only health care providers who can control costs.
    d. Occupational therapists have no impact on case mix analysis.

8. To limit hospital spending, the Federal Government:
   a. Increased retrospective payment rates for Medicare recipients.
   b. Enacted prospective payment rates for Medicare recipients.
   c. Insisted on an increase in length of hospital stay.
   d. None of the above.

9. Which of the following statements is true:
   a. HMOs have decreased in number throughout the U.S.
   b. HMOs cannot negotiate rates for per case reimbursement.
   c. HMOs have grown significantly in recent years.
   d. None of the above.

10. PPOs represent:
    a. The greatest growth area in terms of delivery changes.
    b. A means of controlling health care costs.
    c. a and b.
    d. None of the above.

Answers
1. d
2. d
3. d
4. b
5. d
6. a
7. a
8. b
9. c
10. c

Case Study 1

The occupational therapists in an acute care teaching hospital want to develop their role in the back school program. Specifically, they want to include a session of work simulation for homemaker back problems. The director of OT agreed that this was an important intervention and asked the therapists to provide a cost analysis of this activity.

The therapists must first define the output that is called work simulation. The variable cost of this service was identified as follows:

Output	Time	Wage	Time Cost	Materials Cost	Total Cost
Work Simulation	45 min	.24/min	10.80	.40	11.20

Materials Analysis	Materials	Materials Cost Total		Cost/Individual	Total Cost
Work Simulation	Coffee	Bottle	5.50	.05	
	Milk	Carton	0.50	.05	.40
	Sugar	Packet	0.05	.05	
	Cups	24 cups	2.00	.08	
	Snack	12 servings	2.00		

If the unit cost for occupational therapy is equal to 1 RVU as seen in the example in the chapter and 1 RVU is equal to $3.60, the RVU for work simulation is 3.1. Finally, using the formula in the chapter, the transfer price for this output is $11.20 + $2.10 = $13.10.

Case Study 2

The OT Department at the Rehabilitation Hospital has recently had an increase in referrals for outpatient therapy. The department head must decide how to handle these referrals. The therapists want the hospital to hire more therapists, but the administration does not want to increase the payroll.

The following report is the productivity report for each section of OT for the last four weeks. Based on this report, what should the department head recommend?

The report shows that the inpatient therapists were not meeting the productivity level of 22 units per day. As a result, one therapist will temporarily be transferred to the outpatient area to handle the increase in outpatient referrals. If this increase in referrals continues, the department head must carry out a more detailed cost analysis to determine if an additional staff person should be hired.

Case Study 2
Table A

Productivity Report
Month: June
Section: Inpatient
Therapists: OT
Productivity Standard: 22 units (1 unit = 15 min)

	1	2	3	4	5	6	7	8
	Week	# FTEs allocated/day	# of days	# FTE allocated (2 × 3)	Staff present	Units/Wk	Units/FTE allocated (6-4)	Units/Staff present (6-5)
	4-8	17	5	85	51.0	965	11.4	18.9
	11-15	17	5	85	54.5	941	11.1	17.3
	18-22	17	5	85	54.0	932	11.0	17.3
	25-29	17	5	85	56.8	1027	12.1	18.1

Case Study 2
Table B

Productivity Report
Month: June
Section: Outpatient
Therapists: OT

	1	2	3	4	5	6	7	8
	Week	# FTEs allocated/day	# of days	# FTE allocated (2 × 3)	Staff present	Units/Wk	Units/FTE allocated (6-4)	Units/Staff (6-5)
	4-8	5	5	25	20.0	460	18.4	23.0
	11-15	5	5	25	25.0	583	23.3	23.3
	18-22	5	5	25	22.5	550	22.0	24.4
	25-29	5	5	25	22.5	516	20.1	22.9

References

1. Blosser G, Howells J, McKelvey B, Pierson F. The prospective payment system: its realities and opportunities. *Clin Mgmt.* 5(3):34-44.
2. Coddington DC, Palmquist LE, Trollinger WV. Strategies for survival in the hospital industry. *Harvard Business Rev.* 5:129-133, 1985.
3. Heinemamum AW. Prospective payment for acute care: impact on rehabilitation hospitals. *Arch Phys Med Rehab.* 69(8):614-618, 1988.
4. Home Care, Special Section: *Hospitals* 5/16:64-772, 1985.
5. Logigian MK. Productivity analysis. *Am J Occup Ther.* 41(5):285-291, 1987.
6. Logigian MK, Trisolini MG. A cost analysis and management reporting system in occupational therapy. *Am J Occup Ther.* 41(5):292-296, 1987.
7. Macleod RK. Program budgeting works in nonprofit institutions. *Harvard Business Rev.* 9:46-56, 1971.
8. Marqulies N, Duval J. Productivity management: a model for participative management in health care organizations. *Health Care Management Review* 1(Winter)(6):1-70, 1984.
9. Mistarz JE. Cost accounting: a solution, but a problem. *Hospitals.* 9:96-101, 1984.
10. Orefice JJ, Jennings MC. Productivity—a key to managing cost-per-case. *Health Care Financial Management.* 8:18-24, 1984.
11. Poulsen GP. Detailed costing system nets efficiency, savings. *Hospitals.* 10:106-111, 1984.
12. The Preferred Provider Organization: a response to the environment. *Topics Health Care Financing* Winter:1984.
13. Vladeck BC. Medicare hospital payment by diagnosis related groups. *Ann Intern Med.* 100:576-591, 1984.
14. Woolhandler S, Himmelstein DU. Resolving the cost/access conflict: the case for a national health program. *Journal of General Internal Medicine.* 4:54-60, 1989.

CHAPTER 7

Documentation in Health Care

Janice F. Pagonis, MS, OTR/L

Introduction

In the current health care environment, accurate and timely communication is vital. Although documentation is only one method of communication, it is the most essential component in the delivery of health care services. Today, documentation looks significantly different than it did ten years ago, because of the information explosion and rapid changes in the health care climate. Recent regulations and social pressures greatly altered the quality (content) and the quantity of necessary administrative and clinical recording and reporting in occupational therapy. The prospective payment system for Medicare and Medicaid clients increased the demand for more effective and efficient clinical documentation to justify the need for and the benefit of services. With the present posture of the health care system, knowledge of and skill in documentation are as important as the therapist's clinical and administrative expertise.

Documentation, according to Webster, is "to provide with factual or substantial support for statements made; to equip with exact references to authoritative supporting information."[17] Verification, organization, and standardization of information promotes consistent retrieval and proper utilization of data. In occupational therapy, documentation can be generically categorized as administrative or patient/client related. Samples of administrative documentation are included in this chapter. Some formal administrative documents presented here are mission statements, policies and procedures, reports, proposals, and memorandums. Additionally, administrative documentation can include informal records such as attendance sheets, scheduling forms, and equipment checklists. It is the informal administrative documentation that assists the day-to-day operations. Because of this fact, such informal documents are unique to the individual department and will not be discussed in this chapter.

The second part of the chapter describes health care documentation, which is found in the patient's/client's medical record. It is concerned with the patients/clients and their care. Occupational therapy clinical documentation discussed in this chapter includes initial notes/reports, evaluations/assessment reports, treatment plans, progress notes, and discharge summaries.[4] Documentation in occupational therapy is unique and specific to each facility or service and has a broad scope.

This chapter presents general principles and common forms of basic administrative and clinical documentation. The purpose and elements of recording are discussed and the problem-oriented record is described because it is currently being used by many therapists. The present rules and regulations governing documentation are summarized. This chapter also provides examples from areas such as adult rehabilitation, psychiatry, the school system and home care. This chapter provides only samples, however, because each facility's documentation must meet its own specific needs. Modern trends in documentation can make these examples obsolete. The majority of the regulations presented are those that affect hospital-based services, because the majority of traditional occupational therapy practice is in this setting. Therapists in private practice must be familiar with the rules and regulations of their employers and their regulating and credentialing agencies, and the impact of these regulations on the patient/client population and the third party payors.

Documentation requirements continuously change. The practicing clinician must be aware of the resources available in the health care community on a local, state and federal level and through the American Occupational Therapy Association.

Administrative Documentation

Administrative documentation is any report or statement that facilitates the functions of management and improves departmental operations. These documents are written communiques that organize and coordinate the department/organization and its functions. Administrative documentation varies in style and format. It expresses the values and beliefs of either the author or the institution or both. Most administrative documentation develops from the manager's need to establish organization, coordination, and control in the department. Some of the common administrative documents that are located in the department procedure manual are the departmental philosophy, mission statement, departmental goals/objectives, policies and procedures, and organizational chart. These are specific to each department but might be done at either the departmental or organizational level or both. There are other administrative communiques, such as reports, memorandums, proposals, and notices, which will be discussed in this section.

Philosophy

The philosophy of a department is consistent with that of the institution. The philosophy states the beliefs that give direction to the behaviors of the department. A philosophy is a statement of a value system. It is the theme from which the activities of the department/organization are developed. The undercurrent that leads the vision of the manager comes from the philosophy.

The philosophy is very global, but provides the overall frame of reference for the organizational practice. The philosophical statement of a department varies in length. The beliefs of the theoretical framework on which the department practice is based can be contained in the philosophy (Table 7-1).

Mission Statement

The mission statement or statement of purpose is an extension of the philosophy. The mission statement is general and in a very broad sense answers the question, "Why does this department/organization exist?" It provides a direction for the department. The mission or purpose statement:

- Distinguishes the department/organization from others
- Distinguishes services provided by the department/organization from others
- Specifies the geographic area served
- Identifies the target population
- Is the foundation for establishing goals

A mission statement can be a simple narrative statement or can be expanded in a descriptive outline form. This is dependent on the style of the author and the commitment of the department/organization. The mission statement always remains congruent with the philosophy (Table 7-2).

Goals/Objectives

Goals are broad statements of what is to be accomplished. *Objectives* are derived from the goals. Objectives are specific, measurable statements that can include a time frame and a responsible party. Objectives are more tangible, concrete plans that bring the goals to a practical level. They are often stated as expected outcomes, in behavioral terms. One goal can have many objectives. The goals and objectives provide the direction of the department. Departmental goals and objectives once developed should be reviewed and if necessary, revised on a regular basis or at intervals as part of an ongoing planning process. In participatory management, the entire department is involved in the establishment and

---

Table 7-1
Sample of a Brief Philosophy Statement of an Occupational Therapy Department at a Catholic Hospital

DEPARTMENTAL PHILOSOPHY

The philosophy of the occupational therapy department is consistent with the philosophy of the hospital, which is guided by the teachings of the Roman Catholic Church and the Sisters. It is our belief that all persons are worthy of human dignity and holistic care. Each person is comprised of the body and soul and should be treated as a whole. The principles of charity, which direct the future of the department, preserve the privacy and dignity of the individual, regardless of his/her social or economic status.

completion of the goals and objectives (Table 7-3).

The transition from the philosophy to objectives is an instrumental stage of the planning process. This process creates activities and programs that are guided by a system of beliefs. The planned departmental activity reflects the purpose of the department (Figure 7-1).

Rules and regulations are developed to ensure continued consistency in departmental behavior. Within an organization/department, these rules and regulations are termed policies and procedures. Policies are guidelines to handle recurrent organizational/ departmental problems or a means to avoid potential problems. "Procedures tie all the organizational parts together."[2]

Policy and Procedures

Policies and procedures are the guidelines of action. They state expected behaviors. They promote organization and coordination of services, programs and activities, ensure safety and a level of care. A *policy* is a general statement that outlines an expected course. It might include a rationale and is always approved by the manager and organization. If the policy affects staff in other departments or disciplines, they must be made aware of any changes. The sequential steps in the implementation of the policy are the procedures. *Procedures* support the policy and are the selection of a specific course of action. Procedures answer the questions, "What should be done? How is it to be done?" and, "Who will do it?" Policies and procedures relate to the department's/organization's structure or function. They inform the employee what is expected and what is acceptable. When policies and procedures are clearly and concisely written, they guarantee consistent employee responsibility.

Table 7-2
The Mission or Purpose Statement of Children's Hospital Synthesizes the Commitments of the Departments.

MISSION/PURPOSE STATEMENT

The occupational therapy department of Children's Hospital provides services to those children, from birth to eighteen years of age, with neurological and orthopedic conditions. Direct treatment is provided to both inpatients and outpatients. All services delivered are based on the developmental model.

- Services provided include early intervention and stimulation, physical daily living skills training, sensorimotor learning, developmental activities to promote cognitive and performance skills, therapeutic adaptation, prevention, and family education.
- Consultation is provided to the rehabilitation unit and to the Bay area school district.
- Children's Hospital has limited its services to the area within a (30) thirty mile radius and will send appropriate referrals to other necessary agencies outside this area.
- The department is committed to the highest level of quality care while recognizing the need for efficiency and cost effectiveness.
- Treatment is delivered individually or in groups as determined by the children's needs.

The department further defines its mission to include teaching and training other health care professionals, specifically those in the field of occupational therapy. It is our belief that the services of Children's Hospital directly benefit the community.

Policies and procedures are titled by topic. The policy is then stated succinctly and the procedures are listed in an organized fashion. The advantages, or support of compliance, and the results of noncompliance are stated. Document as policy any rule or information that all staff members are expected to know. Include known expectations or exclusions. Organize these policies and procedures in a manual that is accessible to all staff members. Some institutions provide all staff members with their own policy and procedure handbook while others maintain a handbook in the department. Regardless of the mechanism, all staff are responsible for knowing its contents (Table 7-4).

Organizational Chart

An *organizational chart* is an outline of the formal structure of an organization or department. It is a diagram indicating the formal lines of authority, responsibility, and communication. The diagram consists of lines and boxes. The boxes are *terminals* and represent positions within the department/organization. The lines are called *channels*. They

---

Table 7-3

Samples of the necessary objectives for the goals of instituting a quality assurance plan. Note the broadness of the goal and the specificity of the objectives. The responsible person for each objective is stated.

GOALS/OBJECTIVES

Goal A: To establish a systematic quality assurance program to monitor the quality and appropriateness of care on an ongoing basis. (6 months)

Objective A1: A quality assurance committee will be created from the occupational therapy staff. The director of the department will chair the committee. The committee will include 1 registered occupational therapist, 1 certified occupational therapy assistant, 1 aide and 1 escort. (1 month)

A2: Monthly meetings will be conducted with minutes, recorded by committee secretary, who is elected and approved by the quality assurance committee. (monthly)

A3: The quality assurance committee will develop written protocols that are approved by the occupational therapy staff:
a. Develop draft of protocols. (2 months)
b. Review by staff. (1 month)
c. Revise protocols presented to staff. (3 months)
d. Approved protocols included in department policy and procedures manual. (6 months)

A4: The quality assurance committee will develop and activate a quality of care matrix with appropriate quality monitors. (6 months)

A5: The occupational therapy department will develop a problem list with priorities. (Quality assurance chair will be responsible for the accomplishment of this task.) (6 months)

A6: The proposed system will operate for 3 months and then be assessed on a predetermined criterion by the Quality Assurance Committee. (9 months)

refer to channels of authority, responsibility, and communication. If the channels are solid they indicate a direct relationship between the boxes. Broken lines denote indirect relationships. An indirect relationship can demonstrate a relation specific to a certain task or function. For example, there can be an indirect relationship between the director of occupational therapy of a hospital and the chief executive officer of a community mental health satellite because of contracted service. The relationship might only be concerned with the delivery of a special contracted service and its fiscal responsibility. Figure 7-2 is an example of an organized chart.

When part of a multisystem, the parent corporation and each large facility within the multisystem might have their own organizational chart. Each department within each facility should also have its individual organizational chart to outline the formal lines of authority, responsibility, and communication within the department. Other administrative documents that are often generated by the occupational therapy supervisor as methods of communication are reports, memorandums, and notices.

Reports

Reports are usually produced on a regular basis. Typically there are monthly reports, annual reports, and special reports. Style, length, and content of reports are dictated by the institution or are at the discretion of the occupational therapy manager submitting

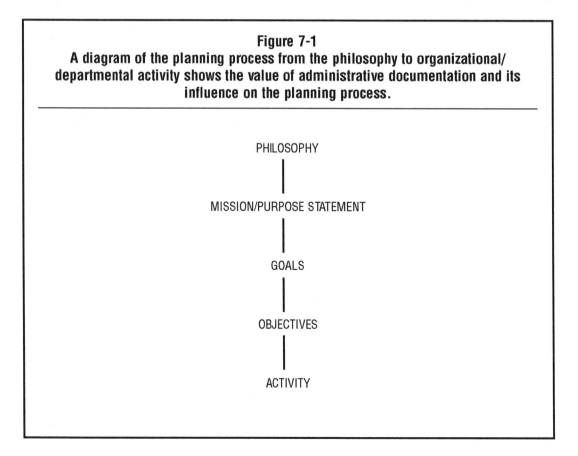

Figure 7-1
A diagram of the planning process from the philosophy to organizational/ departmental activity shows the value of administrative documentation and its influence on the planning process.

PHILOSOPHY

MISSION/PURPOSE STATEMENT

GOALS

OBJECTIVES

ACTIVITY

the report. Monthly reports can include activities of the month, updates on current projects, statistical data, rationale of productivity, achievement of stated goals and plans that were projected for that month, and goals and activities expected to be achieved in the upcoming month. Format is determined by the immediate supervisor of the facility or the facility may have a policy and procedure for the monthly report.

The *monthly report* can be narrative or in an outline form. Monthly reports are submitted to the immediate supervisor to keep this person informed of the activities of the occupational therapy department. If no format is provided, always ask the administrator what should be included in the monthly report and the required deadline.

The *annual report* is a summary of the monthly reports and can include the proposed goals and objectives for the upcoming year. Annual reports can be submitted at the end of the calendar year or the fiscal year. In some institutions, as part of the annual report, the long range planning committee might request a five-year plan. This is a projection of departmental activity.

Table 7-4

A sample policy and procedure for annual staff inservices. This policy consists of title, policy statement, procedures, and result of noncompliance.

POLICY/PROCEDURE
ANNUAL STAFF INSERVICE

Policy	In order to remain current in the areas of safety and employment health, the occupational therapy staff are required to attend the six annual inservices in the areas of: 1. Body mechanics 2. Verbal instruction 3. Fire and safety 4. Electrical safety 5. Infection control 6. Cardiopulmonary resuscitation These inservices are conducted by the staff development department.
Procedures	1. All professionals and occupational therapy staff (OTRs and COTAs) are to attend all six required annual inservices. All nonprofessional staff are excused from the CPR inservice. 2. All occupational therapy staff are responsible for: • Reviewing the monthly education calendar published by the staff development department and posted in the office. • Scheduling attendance at each inservice with the clinical supervisor. • Verifying attendance at each inservice by signing the staff development attendance sheet. • Documenting attendance of each inservice in their individual personnel training profiles, available through the secretary with the date of attendance documented. 3. Noncompliance with this policy will negatively affect annual performance appraisals.

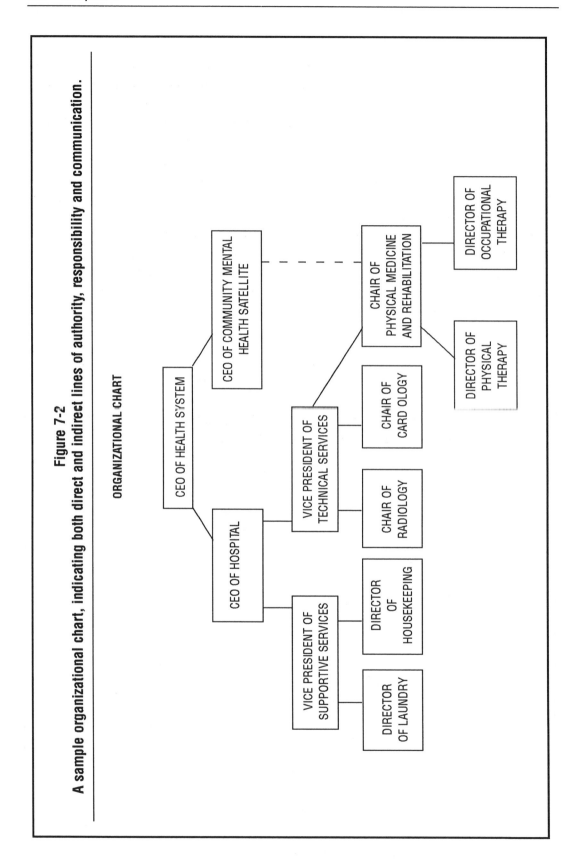

Figure 7-2
A sample organizational chart, indicating both direct and indirect lines of authority, responsibility and communication.

ORGANIZATIONAL CHART

Proposals

A *proposal* is a justification of projected or anticipated programs, personnel, equipment, or space. A proposal is a step-by-step plan of how an idea becomes a reality. For example, when proposing a work hardening program, projections of necessary space, equipment, and personnel are essential. To defend the program, the proposal can include the program goals and objectives, amount and type of treatment, expected revenues (based on the current market) and expenses, and rate of reimbursement. Include any additional start-up costs.

The proposal can include the expected advantages and disadvantages of the planned activity. Some proposal formats include community need or a needs assessment for the service, rationale of program, marketing strategies, physician referral base, and how it differs from current competition. A projected one year budget might be requested.

Memoranda

A *memorandum* or *memo* is a written communication generally utilized to enhance information flow within a system. This paper trail can be beneficial, if used properly. A memo acts as verification that the information was sent, to whom, and when. Make memoranda concise but explicit. The format is simple and the content is directed to a special audience. The "TO" and "FROM" sections indicate the name and title of the sender and the intended receiver. Often "TOPIC" or "RE" (for "regarding") is used to identify the topic of the material. The date is always documented in the heading. Good judgment governs the content of a memo. The information is public once written in a memorandum. A policy of sending a copy of a significant or informational memo to supervisors or other personnel who would benefit from the information is recommended. Many institutions have memo forms printed on the facility's letterhead. Always initial the memorandum. Table 7-5 shows a typical memo.

Notices

Notices may be presented in the memo format and should be typed, dated, and signed. Notices are frequently used to announce new personnel, promotions, events, or a change. A notice should include: what, where, when, and whom. Often the name and the telephone number of a contact person is available for further inquiries (Table 7-6).

The amount and variety of administrative documentation is vast. (Other forms of administrative documentation or methods of recording are covered in other parts of this book.) Although the examples presented in this section might be helpful, it is important to note that administrative documentation is as individual as clinical documentation, greatly influenced by the needs of the facility and the impending rules and regulations. Written communication is a reflection of the individual, whether it is clinical or administrative. Many significant clinical and administrative decisions are based on or influenced by written communication.

Health Care Documentation

Health care documentation is located in the primary health record (medical records, student permanent record) or the secondary health record (departmental files).[15] Both primary and secondary health records are patient and student identifiable. A primary health record is a collection of information related to the individual patient's care and documentation from the health professionals who provided the services. These records are centralized and maintained by the health care facility. The secondary records are the working papers. These can include the actual tests and worksheets. Health care documentation consists of informational data and clinical data. *Informational data* is statistical, demographical, and related to the client's identification, and can include such items as the patient's/client's name, address, and date of admission. Clinical documentation is the recording of clinical data. *Clinical data* is the tracking of the client's course during evaluation and treatment/intervention. Clinical documentation, including the diagnosis or condition, the intervention, and results, is obtained professionally during the course of treatment.[1] Clinical documentation must also include why a patient/client was not seen or

---

Table 7-5
This memo to the vice president is a means to keep him informed and to show appreciation for his interest. By sending a copy to the directors of housekeeping and dietary and the editor of the bulletin, the participation of these departments is reconfirmed. Memos keep the appropriate persons informed.

TO: John Daly, MPH
          Vice President of Ancillary Services
FROM: Paul White, MS, OTR/L
          Director of Occupational Therapy Services
DATE: March 29, 1988
RE: Occupational Therapy Week

Once again it is time to celebrate National Occupational Therapy Week, from April 18th-22nd. As per your suggestion, arrangements have been made for the occupational therapy department to participate in the following activities:

April 18 Monday	Hand Strength Test in the cafeteria 10:00 a.m.-2:00 p.m. Gifts will be awarded to the strongest male and female.
April 19 Tuesday	Information booth in the main lobby, regarding programs at the Medical Center 8:00 a.m.-4:00 p.m.
April 20 Wednesday	Open house for administration and employees in the occupational therapy department 3:00 p.m.-4:00 p.m.
April 21 Thursday	Open house for physicians and their office managers in the occupational therapy department 3:00 p.m.-4:00 p.m.
April 22 Friday	Tours to local high school students to discuss careers in occupational therapy.

Housekeeping and dietary have been involved in the planning and have made excellent suggestions.

cc: D. Cook, Director of Dietary
     M. Clean, Director of Housekeeping

did not participate in therapy. Clinical documentation is extremely important for third party payor reimbursement.

Treatment documentation can be narrative, a checklist, or require completion of an established form. Traditionally, it is hand written, but it can be typed or even computerized, which is the most recent trend. It can be written departmentally or interdisciplinary. How clinical documentation appears varies from setting to setting, and is governed by local, state, and federal laws. Changes in clinical documentation are continuous and are influenced by current trends and the rationale for documentation.

Characteristics of Good Documentation

Although documentation reflects the uniqueness of each facility, there are consistent components of effective documentation. Make sure documentation is organized, clear, concise, complete, accurate, current, objective, and legible. Rules of English composition, correct grammar, and spelling must be used.[4] Use plain and understandable language. Limit the use of professional jargon.[14] Only those symbols and abbreviations approved by the facility are used in writing reports.[13] Include in each entry the date(s) of service and the signature of the therapist.

Always demonstrate good judgment when documenting. Information should not be speculative, judgmental, or misleading. Subjective material or personal opinions, if stated at all, should be indicated as such.

Table 7-6
Notice of announcement of promotion or job change in memo form.

TO: All Department Heads
FROM: Mary Tree, MPH
         Director of Personnel
DATE: May 5, 1988

ANNOUNCEMENT OF NEW DIRECTOR OF SOCIAL SERVICE

Effective Monday, April 25, 1988, Joan Day, MSW, will be the new Director of Social Service. Ms. Day is a graduate of the University of Pittsburgh and has worked at St. Anne Hospital, the Gold Coast Rehabilitation Center, and for the past year has been employed as Assistant Director here at Good Luck Hospital. Ms. Day can be reached at ext. 4789.

Purpose of Recording

The reasons for documentation govern the content and the appearance of the record or report. AOTA outlines the purpose of clinical documentation as to:

1. Provision of a serial and legal record of the patient's condition and the course of the therapeutic intervention from admission to discharge.

2. Service as an information source for patient/client care.
3. Facilitate communication among health care professionals who contribute to the patient's/client's care.
4. Furnish data for use in treatment, education, research, and reimbursement.[4]

Correct documentation ensures the accountability of the professional and validates the care provided. As a legal document, the medical record is retrieved for justification of treatment on which reimbursement decisions are made by third party payors. Legally the records can be subpoenaed by the court to investigate care or substantiate the degree of disability or limitation, or the amount of progress and ability.

Types of Documentation

Most clinical documentation systems include initial reports or evaluations, progress notes, reevaluations, treatment plans, and discharge summaries. Each of these will be described in detail. The *Initial Report,* which can proceed the initial assessment, often contains basic identification and background information. This can be obtained from a variety of sources: referral, medical record, health care professionals, clients, or their guardians. The *Initial Report* usually includes the client's name, age (date of birth), date of referral, referral source, diagnosis, past medical history, precautions or complications, and reason for referral. An initial report or note might only state that the assessment process was started, and why the full evaluation was not completed (Table 7-7).

The *Assessment Note/Evaluation Report* should include the patient's identification information, if not previously stated, the tests or evaluations administered, and the objective findings. An analysis of specific testing tools might be necessary. Standardized tests should be administered when possible and the results reported in the document. Document a brief summary of the results of all other evaluative procedures with a

---

Table 7-7
Sample of an initial note, when patient is not able to be seen. All abbreviations included in this note would be approved by facility.

INITIAL REPORT/NOTE

Patient: Mary Smith
Medical Record No. 024210
3/27/88   Occupational Therapy

Pt. is a 78 y.o. w. ♀ referred on 3/27/88 by Dr. Jones for an ADL evaluation at bedside. Pt. fell on 3/23/88 and sustained an intertrochanteric fracture of left femur. Pt. had an ORIF on 3/24/88. PMH includes DM s/p MI (11/87) and CHF.
Precautions: Cardiac precautions observed; pt. permitted WBAT.
Chart reviewed, but pt. not seen because of scheduling of x-ray and cardiogram. Two unsuccessful attempts were made to see pt. at bedside. Will attempt to see pt. tomorrow.

Janice F. Pagonis, OTR/L

subsequent problem list or recommendations for service.[4] Once the results of the assessment are analyzed, develop long- and short-term goals. Goals are written in consultation with the patient and/or significant others as required by various accrediting agencies. Long-term goals are statements of the expected level of performance at time of patient discharge from the facility or at the conclusion of treatment. They are the desired long-term outcomes. In acute care or hospice care, the long-term goals might cover a short period of time.

Short-term goals are intermediate steps to achieve the long-term goals. Statements of behavioral objectives or expected outcomes might be a necessary part of the assessment note. In the school system, the evaluation report must document educationally related needs provided under PL94-142.[5]

A plan of treatment is proposed based on the goals, with an anticipated time frame for achievement of each goal. This plan of care can be included as part of the assessment process or separated as a specific treatment plan. The development of a *treatment plan* or *plan of care* is usually based on the initial assessment and amended as needed according to reassessments. Comprehensive treatment plans are interdisciplinary or multidisciplinary. A comprehensive treatment plan requires that each treating discipline, including the physician, contribute to one form and initial it. The treatment plan might have columns for a problem list with date of onset, goals, specific objectives, responsible discipline, expected outcome, and anticipated time frame.

A treatment plan summarizes the total management of an individual patient (Figure 7-3). It is updated according to policy and by monitoring the achievement of goals. This document is always dated and signed or initialed by the involved professionals. New goals can be added and others deleted if the client's condition changes. With home care patients, Medicare stipulates a review and appropriate revision of the treatment plan every 60 days. Treatment plans can be compiled by the occupational therapy staff or by the interdisciplinary or multidisciplinary team members.

The *Individual Educational Plan* (IEP) is a treatment plan used in the public school system. It is mandated by PL94-142, The Education for All Handicapped Children Act. Federal regulations state that the IEP must be in effect before special education and related services can be provided to a child.[5] An IEP is completed for each child at least annually. It is based on the initial evaluation, and ideally developed by the treating team members. An IEP contains the following: the child's present status, annual goals and related instructional objectives, expected dates of goal achievement, identification of the services provided, initiation and projected duration of these services, and a schedule for determining, by evaluation, whether the instructional objectives were attained[5] (Table 7-8).

Progress Notes reflect achievement of goals, progress or lack of it, or regression. They generally include treatment/modalities, procedures, and the patient's response to the stated therapeutic intervention. Objective data and subjective perceptions should be indicated as such. Note changes in treatment plans. Expected outcomes are stated as measurable goals, and any necessary recommendations documented. Include the client's frequency of attendance and if the client is consistently absent, briefly explain the reason, if known. The progress note can also report on activities, orthotic devices, equipment, patient/family instruction, and the home exercise program. All progress notes must be signed and dated by

Figure 7-3

A sample of an occupational therapy treatment plan for a home care patient. This departmental plan of care includes the date of onset, problem list, goals, plan, outcome, time frame, and 60-day review. The treatment plan was developed after evaluation on 1/10/88 and at time of 60-day review (3/10/88) achievement of goals noted.

HAPPY HOME CARE AGENCY
TREATMENT PLAN

Date   January 10, 1988

Patient Name   Edward Stroke

Medical Record No.   58-43-19

Diagnosis   (r) CVA with left side paraplegia, hypertension

Discipline   RN_____   OT_____   PT_____   ST_____

Therapist_____

Onset Date	Problems	Goals	Plan/Intervention	Expected Outcome	Time Frame	60-Day Review
11/18/87	1. Dependence in ADLs	1. Improve performance in areas of transfers, bathing, and dressing.	1.a. Transfer-raining	1.a. Patient will be able to transfer from wheelchair to bed, wheelchair to commode, and wheelchair to tub seat with minimal assist of one	2/10/88	Incomplete 3/10/88
			b. ADL in bathing and dressing. Issue necessary adaptive equipment.	b. Patient will require only minimal assistance for set-up for performance of self-care activities.	3/10/88	Incomplete 3/10/88

Figure 7-3 (continued)

Onset Date	Problems	Goals	Plan/Intervention	Expected Outcome	Time Frame	60-Day Review
11/18/87	2. Left side neglect and hemianopsia.	2.a. Increase awareness of left hemibody. b. Improved awareness of left visual field.	2.a. Teach compensatory and protective techniques. b. Teach patient to look to the left.	2.a. Patient will be aware of protective techniques. b. Patient will consistently compensate for visual limitation.	2/10/88 3/10/88	Achieved 3/10/88 Achieved 3/10/88
11/18/87	3. Nonfunctional Left Upper Extremity	3. Increased control and awareness of Left Upper Extremity (LUE)	3. Use facilitatory technique to reduce tone. Gross motor, unilateral and bilateral activities.	3. Patient will be able to use Left Upper Extremity as a stabilizer. Patient will be able to do self-ranging independently.	4/10/88 2/24/88	Partial Achievement 3/10/88 Achieved 3/10/88
1/5/88	4. Depression	4. Involve patient in family activities. Explore avocational interests.	4. Involve family in treatment	4. Patient will eat meals with family at dining room table Patient will play cards using card holder with close friend.	2/10/88 2/10/88	Achieved 3/10/88 Achieved 3/10/88

Table 7-8

An Individual Educational Plan consists of annual goals, related instructional objectives, expected date of completion, service provided, and initiation of services.

INDIVIDUALIZED EDUCATIONAL PLAN

Student's Name:	Patricia Green	School: South Elementary
Birthdate:	4/21/81	Class Placement: Multi-handicapped
Age:	7 years, 7 months	Teacher: Mrs. Apple
Date of IEP:	9/11/88	

Student receives: Speech Therapy _____
                   Occupational Therapy ___X___
                   Physical Therapy ___X___

Annual Goal: (Occupational Therapy)
Improve attentional behaviors.

Short-term objective:

1. Patricia will attend to an activity during treatment for 10 minutes, without asking to end or change the activity, once during each daily treatment session.

Begin: 9/15/88
Complete: 10/15/88
Review: ___/___/___
Achieved: ___/___/___

Comments:

Annual Goal: (Occupational Therapy)
Improve independence in dressing.

Short-Term Objective:

1. Patricia will be able to remove her shoes and socks with minimal assistance at the beginning of the treatment session 3 out of 5 times per week.

Begin: 9/15/88
Complete: 11/15/88
Review: ___/___/___
Achieved: ___/___/___

Comments:

Annual Goal: (Physical therapy)
Improve ambulation on stairs.

Short-term Objective:

1. Patricia will be able to ascend stairs with a minimum of ten steps, independently with spotting, 80% of the time.

Begin: 9/15/88
Complete: 12/15/88
Review: ___/___/___
Achieved: ___/___/___

Comments:

the therapist responsible for the individual patient. Student's notes must be countersigned by the supervising therapist.

When a patient is discontinued from occupational therapy services, write a *Discharge Summary* or report. Do this report as close as possible to the time of patient discharge, so that information is accurate and available to all health professionals in a timely manner. There is usually a departmental policy regulating the timeliness of the discharge summary. The discharge report is a summary of the delivery of services. It generally compares the status of the patient at discharge with that patient's functional performance during the initial evaluation. It also includes the number of treatments or visits, the reason for discontinuation of services, and the disposition of the patient. Discussion of the achievement or lack of achievement of the established long- and short-term goals is included in the discharge report, with the date of discharge or last day of treatment indicated.[4] This report also includes any discharge instructions, home programs and recommendations, and summarizes any equipment or orthotic devices issued. If a follow-up evaluation or appointment is scheduled, document the date and purpose of appointment. Include in the summary a referral to any other agency or community service.

The Problem-Oriented Record

Notewriting has changed throughout the years based on current trends and the demands of health care. Brief and infrequent notes have developed into descriptive and lengthy narratives. The style of documentation is dictated by the needs of the facility. A recent and widely used format of documentation in the 1980s is the problem-oriented approach. The value of the problem-oriented system is that it is organized, logical, and efficient. The four basic elements of the problem-oriented record, as proposed by Weed,[18] are data base, problem list, plan and progress notes.

The data base includes the identification and background information, chief complaint, and results of the assessment by each of the participating team members. From this data, a current problem list is created and the problems numbered. If additional problems develop during the course of care, they are numbered consecutively and added to the list. A *treatment plan* or *plan of care* is a component of the problem-oriented system. The treatment plan includes the proposed interventions associated with each numbered problem on the original problem list. A treatment plan generally includes the following categories: problem list, date of onset of problem, goals/objectives, intervention, responsible discipline/party and anticipated time frame to achieve expected outcome. Figure 7-4 shows an example of a treatment plan.

All documentation in the treatment plan deals with the solution of the problems listed. This style of modern documentation promotes an efficient, effective, yet objective data base system. The progress notes gather current ongoing information and the results of treatment intervention. Progress notes can be handled as a flow sheet where applicable. In problem-oriented medical records, each progress note has a relationship to a numbered problem. For example, if poor self-image is problem number 3, a progress note discussing the

Figure 7-4

This is a sample of a problem-oriented system with the progress note relating to the problem list in the treatment plan.

INTERDISCIPLINARY TREATMENT PLAN

Patient ___Suzie Q___

Diagnosis ___Depression___

Date ___4/15/88___

Medical Record No. ___320124___

Physician ___Dr. Way___

Date	Problem Letter	Problem Statement	Goals	Objective	Discipline	Time Frame
4/15/88	A	Limited self-expression A_1 Limited verbalization to authority figures or in group	A_1 Able to verbalize feelings to psychiatrist, nurses, and in group situations	A_1 Client able to personalize and communicate feelings of anger to psychiatrist in private session $3 \times$ in $1/2$ hr. session	RN OT SS RT	4/22/88
				Client able to initiate conversation in group $3 \times$ in 1 hr. session.	MD	4/22/88
		A_2 Rigid body posture	A_2 Able to allow consistent expression of self through body movements as well as verbalization	A_2 Client able to consistently express congruence in body movements with specific emotional and competitive situations	RN OT SS RT	4/22/88
				Client able to verbalize feelings appropriately	RN OT RT SS	4/22/88
	B	Poor self-concept	B Patient will recognize self-worth	B_1 Client will refer to self in a positive manner	RN OT RT	
				B_2 Patient will exhibit good hygiene and self-care habits	RN OT	
				B_3 Patient will recognize and take pride in her accomplishments	RN OT RT	

Figure 7-4 (continued)

Patient   Suzie Q

Medical Record No.   320124   Date   4/22/88

Progress Note

 # A S: "It's hard for me to say what I want to say."

     "It felt funny and good to say what I felt like saying."

O: In group session, client was able to initiate conversation without prompting 5 ×. Client expressed anger at mother's behavior. Client was able to sustain eye contact with 4 out of 5 of the group members 80% of the group session.

A: Client appeared uncomfortable and expressed self-satisfaction in being able to talk within the group.

LONG-TERM GOAL: Client will comfortably express feelings and needs consistently in all situations.

SHORT-TERM GOALS: (1) Client will initiate conversation in group situation.

                         (2) Client will express pride in her completion of tasks and positive feelings of self and abilities.

P: Client will be scheduled for movement group and general activity group to allow physical expression of feelings.

client's performance in a 'Hygiene Group' would be numbered 3.

The advantages of the problem-oriented record are:

1. A note is not written unless there is data to record.
2. The format provides the opportunity for self-evaluation as well as peer evaluation.
3. It allows data that supports the need for occupational therapy services to be collected.
4. It provides a clear description of the patient's condition and rehabilitative potential.
5. It is possible to state specifically what service was delivered and the results of the service.[6]

An adaptation of the Weed method is commonly called *SOAP* note writing. S-O-A-P is an acronym for subjective, objective, assessment, and plan. This can be done with or without a relationship to an original problem list. The *subjective* section includes any information that is subjective, which is what the patient communicates to the therapist. This is often a direct quote from the patient. The subjective section can include the patient's feelings, complaints, goals, home environment, or available resources. The *objective* portion of the SOAP note is a demonstrated level of performance, results of reevaluation or tests, and concrete reports. The *assessment* is always based on the objective data and summarizes the client's strengths and weaknesses. The assessment portion connotes the present condition, progress, change, and justification for treatment. The assessment area can include the client's level of participation and motivation. The *plan* section includes treatment goals, long-term and short-term goals. In other systems, the short-term and long-term goals can be included in the plan section. The plan would be the therapist's recommendations and follow-up care. The time and frequency of any follow-up care should be in the plan portion of the SOAP note. The plan should logically succeed the assessment. Kuntavanish[9] adds pre-SOAP and post-SOAP steps. The pre-SOAP procedure involves reading available chart information, physician evaluation, past medical history, past performance, and pre-hospitalization record. The post-SOAP is a discharge summary or follow-up reevaluation.

A Professional Responsibility

Documentation and confidentiality are professional responsibilities supported by *The Principles of Occupational Therapy Ethics*.[12] These principles guide professional conduct in the field and direct occupational therapists to conform to local, state, and federal laws and regulations applicable to records and reports. Occupational therapists are obligated to record information as required by the standards of both the employer and AOTA. When conflict or differences arise among these standards, regulations, or laws, the occupational therapist is responsible for reporting these discrepancies to the employer. This responsibility includes monitoring the corrective action. The occupational therapist is responsible for her/his own behavior as determined by the principles. The principles also clearly state that objective data shall govern subjective data in evaluations, recommendations, records, and reports.[12] Objective data has influenced the credibility of the profession since it provides a means of health accountability. Objective and precise records are a mechanism that relates outcome to therapeutic intervention.[10] The reporting process presents the merits of occupational therapy to the client, third party payor, physician and other health care professionals.[3]

The privacy and confidentiality of client information is only addressed by the profession's Code of Ethics and the Rights and Responsibilities of the patient section of the Joint Commission on Accreditation of Healthcare Organizations (JCAHO) manuals, and the Federal Privacy Act of 1974.[15] The occupational therapist has the responsibility to utilize all related information solely for the improvement of the client's well-being and safety. To guarantee confidentiality, some states have laws specifically addressing defamation, slander, libel, disclosure of information, and privacy. The Privacy Act of 1974 permits clients or their representatives to review the client's medical record in a federal hospital or agency upon request. In addition, the act also allows clients or their representatives to appeal for changes or corrections of the medical records.[14]

The patient's bill of rights grants all patients/clients the right to see information in their records. The patient must have a legitimate reason for wanting to view the chart and it is generally recommended that the physician or appropriate health care professional be available to clarify the information. Certain states have statutes regarding this right and various institutions have developed their own patient bill of rights.[15] The therapist should be familiar with this document and remember to use good judgment when writing in the medical record. Release of the client's clinical information to outside agencies must be authorized by the client or a legal guardian. A signed authorization sanctions the release of the client's medical information related to the diagnosis, condition, or treatment to outside sources. Generally, medical release forms are available through the medical records department. If a separate release authorization form is designed, it should include what specific information can be released, to who, for what purpose, and for how long the release is effective. The form must be signed by the client or guardian.

Charting for Clinical Research

More and more treatment documentation is being used by third party payors to justify professional intervention based on clinical change. Simple clinical performance can be charted and compared to other subjects by the use of operational definitions and proper recording. Accurate observations and measurements can support and demonstrate the benefits of therapeutic intervention. The use of operational definitions, standardized treatment procedures, and proper documentation enable therapeutic interventions to be monitored and compared. The more specific and accurate the clinician's records, the more replicable the treatment.[10] Relationships can be made between clinical intervention and outcome. Charts, graphs, or flow charts can often monitor clinical change accurately. For example, the performance on the Bartel Index of those patients/clients with Parkinsonism on trial doses of specific medications can be graphed during the rehabilitative process and a possible relationship between the medication level and function established.

Statistical, demographic, and factual data can be studied, as long as the confidentiality of the subject is maintained.[15] The clinic or treatment area is an enriched environment for data collection and data that can ensure accountability. Clinical documentation that is systematic and objective can demonstrate the efficacy of a therapeutic procedure. When documentation systems are similar, they allow comparison among facilities and various patient populations. If documentation is located in the primary health record, data can be retrieved for purposes such as education and research. Often the retrieval of such information is facilitated by medical record personnel.

Documentation Rules and Regulations

There are specific rules and regulations that control clinical documentation in the medical record. Often these requirements are developed by regulating agencies and supported by the medical records department, institution and professional organizations.

Include the client's name and identification number on every page of documentation. The professional's signature should minimally contain first and last name, and professional designation (i.e., OTR/L, COTA/L, OTS, OTAS).[4] AOTA, in the Guidelines for Documentation,[4] states that a registered occupational therapist countersigns all student reports and those of certified occupational therapy assistants if this is required by the employer or legislation. Often the rules and regulations of a licensure board or institution will require cosigning of notes to indicate some level of supervision.

Black ink is used for all handwritten documents to aid duplication and ensure permanence. The medical records department might mandate a specific correction procedure for errors made in the primary health record. Erasing or 'whiting out' is not permissible. The error is never erased, or covered, but instead a line is drawn through the mistake, which is enclosed in parentheses. The word 'error' is written above the mistake and the change is initialed. When documentation is electronic or automated, the use of a computer code or initials is as legal as a written signature for identification or authentication.[15]

Increasingly, compliance with the standards of accrediting and licensing agencies is the motivator for comprehensive documentation. Some of the current minimal regulations affecting documentation in various settings are included in Figure 7-5. Each accrediting agency publishes its own standards or rules and generally these are updated annually. Compliance with these rules and regulations are what the individual surveyors assess when they visit a facility. A manual frequently used by the occupational therapy community is the *Accreditation Manual for Hospitals and Long-Term Care Standards*. Medicare and Medicaid guidelines and changes are generally published in the *Federal Register* and distributed to the local intermediaries within the individual states. With accrediting agencies, vague or general standards are subject to the interpretation of the individual surveyors. Surveyors should be used as resources when questions arise regarding standards. It is essential that therapists delivering health care be knowledgeable of the current documentation standards including those of the national accrediting and licensing agencies as well as those of the federal, state, and local government.

If treatment information is used in research, it must not contain any identifiable data. When using patients for clinical studies in which normal treatment is withheld or

Figure 7-5

Regulations as stated in the 1985 Long-Term Care Manual, the 1988 Accrediting Manual for Hospitals and the Guidelines for Occupational Therapy Services.

	Initial Evaluation	Progress Notes	Plan of Care	Discharge Summary
HOSPITALS (PHYSICAL REHABILITATIVE SERVICES)	— Functional assessment with evidence of participation of patient and family in goal setting. — Measurable goals are described in functional or behavioral terms with frames.	— Progress assessed on timely basis: At least monthly for outpatients and at least every two weeks for inpatients. — Document patient's progress and response to treatment. — If appropriate, revise treatment goals.	— Treatment plan relates to achieve stated goals.	
COMMISSION ON ACCREDITATION OF REHABILITATION FACILITIES	— Clinical information should be recorded within 48 hours of the event. — Includes referring source. — Must be signed and dated by competent professionals. — Includes evidence of individual's participation in the decision-making process of his/her program. — Includes short- and long-term goals. — Current diagnosis. — Findings.	— Include individual treatment plans. — Ongoing assessment of appropriateness of care. — Review of individual program and goals. — Document change in individual's plan for services, goals or treatment techniques.	— Includes patient's rehabilitation problem. — Goals. — Treatment or service provided. — Specific service goals. — Time interval of outcome review. — Anticipated time frame of achieved goals. — Measures to be used to assess effect of treatment/service. — Persons responsible for plan implementation.	— Must be recorded within two weeks following discharge. — Include whether rehabilitative goals achieved an outcome.

Figure 7-5 (continued)

	Initial Evaluation	Progress Notes	Plan of Care	Discharge Summary
LONG TERM CARE (REHABILITATIVE SERVICES)	— Evaluate each patient/resident referred for service. — Recommending a rehabilitative treatment regimen for patient referred. — Assessment of each patient/resident's rehabilitation potential and functional maintenance needs.	— Re-evaluating the patient/resident's continuing need for the service and consulting with the attending physician. — Documentation in progress notes of the provision of and response to rehabilitative services.	— A multidisciplinary plan of care for each patient/resident — Review and revision, as necessary, of those aspects of the multidisciplinary plan of care that pertain to the patient/resident's rehabilitation care.	
HOME CARE SERVICES (REHABILITATIVE SERVICES)	— Each patient receives an initial evaluation to determine the appropriateness of the patient's health care needs for home care services. — Due one week after visit/service.	— Due one week after visit/service. — Signed and dated. For each visit include: a. treatments. b. change in condition. c. patient/family education. d. a summary statement.	Refers to: — All patient diagnoses. — The prognosis, including the short term and long term objectives of treatment. — The types and frequency of services to be provided, including any medication, diet treatment, procedures, equipment, and transportation required. — The functional limitations of the patient. — The activities permitted. — The safety measures required to protect the patient from injury. — Not less than once every 60 days.	— Include summary statement, disposit and if applicable, referral to other services.

Figure 7-5 (continued)

	Initial Evaluation	Progress Notes	Plan of Care	Discharge Summary
SCHOOL SYSTEM	— Vary with school system. — Must have parental consent to test child for preplacement evaluation.		Individual Education Plan (IEP) for each child shall include: "— a statement of present level of performance. — annual goals including short-term instructional objectives. — specific special education and related services and the child's ability to participate in regular education program. — the projected dates for initiation of services and the anticipated duration of services. — appropriate objective criteria and evaluation procedures and schedule for determining, on at least an annual basis, whether the short-term instructional objectives are being achieved."[5]	
COMPREHENSIVE OUTPATIENT REHABILITATION FACILITIES (MEDICARE GUIDELINES)	Includes: — physician referral — diagnosis — requested treatment — date of onset of injury — date of referral — patient's rehabilitation potential or prognosis — short-term/long-term goals in behavioral terminology.		Be included in note.	

experimental treatment provided, the patients or their families must be informed and an agreement or informed consent of participation is required.

Storage and retention of primary health records are strictly controlled, especially if handled by a medical records department. Medical records departments are knowledgeable about federal and state standards and laws relating to the storage, retention, and organization of these records. State statues stipulate various lengths of record retention and permissibility of microfilming records. The therapist in private practice or who owns a private agency that is responsible for the retention of the primary health care record must be cognizant of these laws. Also, the therapist who is responsible for a medical record or any part of the original health record needs to protect these records as a professional responsibility. Health records must be protected against loss, defacement, and tampering and from use by unauthorized individuals.[7]

Use of Medical Records

When discussing clinical documentation, the importance of the medical records department as a resource should not be overlooked. The medical records personnel are familiar with the current regulations regarding the storage and retention of the primary record. There are strict rules that govern the care of primary records. Original records in the primary health record must be kept for three years and then can be microfilmed. The American Hospital Association recommends that primary health records be maintained for 15 years, unless otherwise dictated by state statute.[15]

Although traditionally clinical documentation is handwritten, the more recent trend is to computerize or automate the information. Before a form or format is to become part of the client's primary health care record, it necessitates approval from a forms committee, which usually includes a representative from the medical records department.

Computers and data base systems might influence the future of documentation. These systems have the capacity to improve timely and accurate entries, but comprehensiveness and detail might be sacrificed.

The information in the medical record is essential to the care provided. Not only is the medical record the legal communication among the treating professionals and physician, it is scrutinized by third party payors to determine reimbursement potential. Third party payors rely on the reports to substantiate whether appropriate care was provided to justify the benefit of ongoing care, need for additional care, and that the prescribed care was medically necessary. The utilization review committee examines the charts to determine proper utilization of services and whether a patient continues to need the specialized care of the individual institution. The organization's quality assurance committees should be able to monitor patient progress or the lack of it, achievement of established goals, and even the therapist clinical competence through documentation. Valid documentation can permit comparison of therapeutic approaches and the results of therapeutic intervention by notations of clinical change. Objective and measurable data supporting clinical change can also be used for clinical education, research, and a system for establishing accountability.[11]

A Documentation System

When developing or upgrading a documentation system, many factors must be considered. All components of the system should complement one another. The initial note should relate to the referral. The discharge summary should be a compendium of the initial assessment, progress note, and treatment plan. Similarities should be visible within the system. The question, "What is the purpose of this documentation?" should always be asked. Another question is, "Does there need to be specific areas outlined in the documentation protocols or on the evaluation note format?" (Table 7-9).

A documentation system should be congruent with the philosophy of the department. If a department followed neurodevelopmental frame of reference, the discharge summary would not include a section on orthotic devices. AOTA has developed guidelines for documentation and these should be considered when developing a documentation system. Proper identification and background information should be presented. The system can include a mechanism to convey initial assessment and reassessment, treatment planning, treatment implementation, and discontinuation of services. Is uniform terminology incorporated into the system? Are the fundamental elements of documentation present? (Table 7-10).

The documentation system should be in compliance with departmental and institutional policy. The documentation forms must follow the approved format and must be uniform throughout the facility. If abbreviations are on the form, they must be accepted by the facility. All the reports in the medical record should have prior approval from the facility. Also consider outside regulations (State Health Department, federal, state, and local legislation: JCAHO, CARF, school districts, and third party payors).

Table 7-9
The ten elements of documentation as presented in the American Occupational Therapy Association's *Guidelines for Occupational Therapy Documentation*

1. Patient's full name and case number on each page of documentation.
2. Date stated as month, day, and year for each entry.
3. Identification of type of documentation and department name.
4. Signature with a minimum of first name, last name, and designation.
5. Signature of recorder directly at the end of the note without space left between the body of the note and the signature.
6. Countersignature by a registered occupational therapist (OTR) on documentation written by students and/or certified occupational therapy assistants (COTA) if required by law or facility.
7. Compliance with confidentiality standards.
8. Acceptable terminology as defined by the facility.
9. Facility approved abbreviations.
10. Errors corrected by drawing a single line through the error and the correction initialed (liquid correction fluid and/or erasures are not acceptable), or facility requirements followed.

In addition, can the system foster use of data retrieved for education, research, and quality assurance? When all of these factors are weighed and an appropriate system is developed, the departmental policies should include each component of the system in a clear and specific manner. Objectivity, accuracy, and brevity without sacrifice of essential facts remain the hallmarks of effective recording. The challenge then is the development of a comprehensive and efficient system of documentation that meets the needs of the individual department, institution, and third party payors, complies with all requirements, and still allows the therapist time for quality patient care.

Table 7-10
These questions should be asked when designing or
revising a documentation system.

CONSIDERATIONS FOR A DOCUMENTATION SYSTEM

1. Is the system consistent with the philosophy of the organization/department?
2. Does the system meet the needs of the organization/department?
3. Does the documentation system comply with the standards or rules of the external regulating agencies?
4. Is the system approved by medical records, the forms committee, or any necessary internal committee?
5. Does the system conform to the 'guidelines of documentation' by the American Occupational Therapy Association?
6. Does the system document sufficient information to justify treatment?
7. Is the system readily usable by other health care professionals?
8. Does the system allow retrieval of information for education and research?
9. Are the abbreviations used in the system approved by the medical records department?
10. Does the system utilize uniform terminology?

Questions

1. A department philosophy is:
    a. A statement of purpose
    b. A belief system that gives direction to the department
    c. A general statement of "why the department exists"
    d. A broad statement of "what is to be accomplished"
    e. None of the above

2. The mission statement or statement of purpose:
    a. Is the foundation for establishing goals
    b. Describes the services provided and the target population
    c. Specifies the geographic area served
    d. All of the above
    e. a and b only

3. An organizational chart:
    a. Is made up of terminal and channels
    b. Is a diagram demonstrating the informal lines of authority, responsibility, and communication
    c. Represents direct and indirect organizational relationships by solid and broken lines
    d. All of the above
    e. a and c only

4. Which of the following are different types of reports?
    a. Special reports
    b. Annual reports
    c. Long range planning reports
    d. Monthly reports
    e. a, b, and d

5. Health care documentation:
    a. Consists of both informational and clinical data
    b. Is patient-related
    c. Is located on both the primary and secondary records
    d. All of the above
    e. a and b only

6. Some of the characteristics of good documentation include:
    a. The language should be plain and understandable
    b. Each entry should be signed and dated
    c. The content should be clear, concise, complete, accurate, objective, and legible
    d. The content should contain limited use of professional jargon
    e. All of the above

7. An initial report differs from an assessment note/evaluation report because:
    a. It need not contain the results of the evaluation
    b. It usually includes the client's name, age, date of referral
    c. It is signed and dated by the therapist
    d. b and c only
    e. a and c only

8. A treatment plan or plan of care contains all of the following except:
    a. Problem list
    b. Results of assessment
    c. Date of onset
    d. Goals of treatment/expected outcome
    e. Responsible discipline

9. As proposed by Weed, the problem-oriented record:
    a. Is organized, logical and efficient
    b. Contains four basic elements: data base, the problem list, the plan, and the progress note
    c. Includes "pre-soap" and "post-soap" note writing
    d. All of the above
    e. a and b only

10. Clinical documentation is used by:
    a. Third party payors to recommend reimbursement
    b. Researchers and educators to collect data
    c. Quality assurance committees to assess clinical practice and investigate quality care issues
    d. Lawyers to provide substantiating information to support litigation
    e. All of the above

Answers
1. b
2. d
3. e
4. e
5. d
6. e
7. a
8. b
9. e
10. e

Case Study 1
Administrative Documentation

As the manager of the occupational therapy department of a small non-profit, Catholic community hospital, all of your current administrative documentation is congruent with the philosophy and beliefs of Holy Ghost Hospital, Sisters of Mercy, and teachings of the Roman Catholic Church. Because of these values, the surrounding health care facilities frequently referred the care of the elderly, unemployed, and indigent to Holy Ghost Hospital.

This burden of care became too great for Holy Ghost Hospital to bear after the impact of the prospective payment system, and in the economically depressed "Steel Valley." With the demise of the steel industry, the youth of the area left the Valley to find gainful employment. This left only the unemployed, retired, sick, and poor. At this time, Holy Ghost Hospital was the major employer in the Steel Valley community. The recent shortage of health care professionals added to the staffing problems.

Because of many factors, including fiscal overextension, Holy Ghost Hospital was sold to a national health care management firm, Management Consolidation. Management Consolidation has an excellent reputation for the efficient and effective provision of quality care. They are business oriented and they believe that each individual is responsible for his/her care and that prevention and patient/community programs are essential to maintaining the individual's awareness. Management Consolidation believes that quality health care can be provided by qualified health care workers using sound business principles to create a profit.

This change of ownership will necessitate significant changes in current administrative documentation. The philosophy and mission statement(s) of the facility and individual departments will need to include the for profit emphasis, business orientation, and shift to patient/individual responsibility. The goals and objectives will reflect this new philosophy and might include development of community and patient education programs which will facilitate health maintenance.

The organizational chart of Holy Ghost Hospital will reflect the new corporate structure. There might even be a change in the departmental organizational chart, specifically to whom the occupational therapy manager reports. Level of management and supervision might be affected. Staffing might change. Aides and assistants positions might replace registered therapists positions.

Alterations of the philosophy/mission statement(s), goals and objectives, programming, and organizational structure would impact present policies and procedures. Policies and procedures would ensure increased fiscal responsibility. Patients might be required to purchase expensive adaptive equipment instead of having these items provided as billed items. Corporate change has a "ripple effect" on department management and clinical practice.

Case Study 2
Clinical Documentation

Mr. Joy is 48 years old and works as a bartender. He has a history of hypertension, which has been treated with medication for the past 7 years. On July 8, 1988, he went to his oral surgeon to have a tooth removed under anesthesia. Following the surgery, he had a sudden onset of right side weakness and slurred speech. He was admitted to Good Samaritan Hospital on that day and was referred by Dr. Good on July 10 for occupational therapy, bedside, for evaluation and treatment. The occupational therapist reviewed the medical chart and discovered that Mr. Joy is married and has two children: a 7-year-old son and an 11-year-old daughter. He and his wife live in a ranch home in Springville.

The physician and nursing notes state that he is an insulin-dependent diabetic and that presently Mr. Joy requires moderate assistance to bathe, dress himself, and transfer out of bed into a chair. After the medical chart was reviewed, the occupational therapist heads for Mr. Joy's room. She enters the room, introduces herself, and explains what occupational therapy is and what she will be doing. As she begins the initial assessment, a litter is wheeled into the room by the nurses. "The patient is scheduled for a CAT scan of the brain."

Because the therapist spent time reviewing the medical records and an initial contact was made, an initial report is documented. The initial report includes relevant medical/social information, additional data from the interview and findings of the initial assessment. Why the evaluation was not completed or when it will be completed can be stated briefly. The initial report is part of the permanent medical record.

Even though the patient was seen briefly, the therapist can begin developing a problem list for the occupational therapy treatment plan. Some problems might include: limited function in right upper extremity, moderate assistance in activities of daily living, and loss of current life roles (father, husband, and breadwinner). When the assessment is completed, the comprehensive problem list developed and appropriate goals and expected outcomes determined, a treatment plan can be formulated. The treatment plan includes the plan or intervention and a projected time frame.

Initial Project—Sample

Mr. Joy is a 48-year-old black male admitted on 7/8/88 c̄ right side weakness and slurred speech. PMH includes hypertension, insulin-dependent diabetes mellitus. Patient was referred by Dr. King on 7/10/88 for an occupational therapy evaluation and treatment at bedside. Medical chart was reviewed and nursing notes report patient requires moderate assistance for ADLs.

Patient seen initially at bedside. Patient was alert, oriented × 3, and cooperative. Patient's speech was slow and deliberate. Verbal responses were delayed; apparent word finding difficulty noted. Evaluation interrupted because of medical test. Patient requires moderate assistance of one to transfer from supine to lying to sitting on bed edge. Static sitting balance fair. Patient requires moderate assistance of one to transfer from bed side to wheelchair using stand pivot technique.

Patient will be scheduled tomorrow for completion of evaluation.

Case Study 2
Occupational Therapy Treatment Plan/Care Plan

Date of Onset	Problem	Goal	Intervention Therapy	Expected Outcome	Time Frame
7/8/88	RUE function	AROM Muscle strength	Facilitory techniques Functional activities	Patient will be able to use RUE as an assistive UE	9/8/88
		Gross and fine coordination	Bilateral gross and fine motor activities	Patient will be able to independently follow home exercise program	7/17/88
7/8/88	Fair static sitting balance	Good static sitting balance	Balance activities in sitting position	Patient will have good static and dynamic sitting balance	8/8/88
7/8/88	Limited ADLs	I in self-care with assistive devices	Self care training using appropriate adaptive devices	Patient will be I in self-bathing, feeding, and dressing using special techniques and devices	8/8/88
		Improve ability to transfer	Balance activities	Patient will require minimal assistance for transfers	8/8/88

References

1. Bruce JC. *Privacy and Confidentiality of Health Care Information*. Chicago: American Hospital Association. 1984.
2. Ford RC, Heaton CP. *Principles of Management: A Decision-Making Approach*. Virginia: Reston Publishing Company, 1980.
3. Gillette NP. Nationally Speaking: A Data Base for Occupational Therapy Documentation Through Research. *Am J Occup Ther*. 36(8):499-501, August, 1982.
4. Guidelines for Occupational Therapy Documentation. *Am J Occup Ther*. 40(12):830-832, December, 1986.
5. *Guidelines for Occupational Therapy in the School System*. Rockville: American Occupational Therapy Association, 1987.
6. Hopkins HL, Smith HD (eds): *Willard and Spackman's Occupational Therapy* (5th Ed.) Philadelphia: J.B. Lippincott, 1983.
7. Joint Commission on Accreditation of Hospitals. *Accrediting Manual for Hospitals*. Chicago: Joint Commission of Accreditation of Hospitals, 1988.
8. Joint Commission of Accreditation of Hospitals. *Long-Term Care Standards Manual*. Chicago: Joint Commission of Accreditation of Hospitals, 1985.
9. Kuntavanish A. *Occupational Therapy Documentation: A System to Capture Outcome Data for Quality Assurance and Program Promotion*. Rockville: The American Occupational Assurance and Program Promotion.
10. Ottenbaucher K. *Evaluating Clinical Change: Strategies for Occupational and Physical Therapists*. Baltimore: Williams & Wilkins, 1986.
11. Ottenbaucher K, Johnson MB, Hojem M. The Significance of Clinical Change and Clinical Change of Significant: Issues and Methods. *Am J Occup Ther*. 42(3):156-163, March, 1988.
12. *Principles of Occupational Therapy Ethics*. Rockville: The American Occupational Therapy Association, Adopted 1977 (Revised 1980).
13. Skurka MF, Converse ME (eds.) *Organization of Medical Records Departments in Hospitals*. Chicago: American Hospital Association, 1984.
14. Society for Hospital Social Worker Directors. *Documentation by Social Workers in Medical Records*. Chicago: American Hospital Association, 1984.
15. Springer EW. *Automated Medical Records and the Law*. Rockville: Aspen System Corporation, 1971.
16. *Standards Manual for Organizations Serving People with Disabilities*. Arizona: Commission on Accreditation of Rehabilitation Facilities, 1987.
17. *Webster's New Collegiate Dictionary*. Massachusetts: G & C Merriam Company, 1981.
18. Weed LL. *Medical Records, Medical Education and Patient Care*. Chicago: The Press of Case Western Reserve, 1970.

CHAPTER 8

Designing Fieldwork Programs

Ellen S. Cohn, EdM, OTR/L, FAOTA

Introduction

Historically, the practical or fieldwork components of our education are rooted in the philosophical notion that education for professionals is both theoretical and practical.[15] As we survey the literature we find support for the assertion that fieldwork continues to function as the lynchpin between the academic world of theory and the clinical world of practice. "Fieldwork is intended to complement academic preparation by offering additional opportunities for growth, for learning to apply knowledge, for developing and testing clinical skills, and for validating and consolidating those functions that comprise professional competence."[12] The value of the fieldwork experience was documented by Christie, Joyce, and Moeller who surveyed students and supervisors in 65 fieldwork centers. They found that fieldwork had the greatest impact on the development of a therapist's preference for a specific area of clinical practice.[5] Today, the fieldwork experience continues to serve as a critical component of our professional education.

Purpose of Fieldwork Education

This component of our education functions as the gateway into our profession because all students must complete this phase of their professional preparation in order to become eligible to take the certification examination for occupational therapists and occupational therapy assistants. In addition to academic course work, AOTA *Essentials and Guidelines of an Accredited Educational Program for the Occupational Therapist* and *Essentials and Guidelines of an Approved Educational Program for the Occupational Therapy Assistant* require two levels of fieldwork experience for all occupational therapy students.[1] This chapter will define the levels of fieldwork experiences recognized by the AOTA, the roles and responsibilities of the key players, and present a framework for deciding whether to establish a fieldwork education program. Additionally, the chapter will provide the occupational therapy manager with the foundation to develop a fieldwork program.

Levels of Fieldwork Experience

Level I fieldwork offers students practical experiences that are integrated throughout the academic program. The overall purpose of the Level I fieldwork experience is to provide students with exposure to clinical practice through observation of clients and therapists. Through these observations students have the opportunity to examine their reactions to clients, themselves, other personnel, and the profession. Because the academic level, performance expectations, and specific purpose of the Level I fieldwork experience vary throughout each occupational therapy curricula, the timing, length, requirements, and specific focus of the Level I fieldwork experience are negotiated with each academic program on an individualized basis.

Level II fieldwork is designed to "promote clinical reasoning and reflective practice; to transmit the values, beliefs and ethical commitments of the field of occupational therapy, to communicate and model professional behaviors attending to the developmental nature of career growth and responsibility; and to develop and expand a repertoire of occupational therapy assessments and treatment interventions related to human performance." The requirements established by the AOTA include a minimum of six months of Level II fieldwork experience for occupational therapy students and a minimum of two months for occupational therapy assistant students. To offer students "experience with a wide range of client ages and a variety of physical and mental health conditions," the six months are usually divided into two three-month experiences in different clinical facilities. Some academic programs require an extra three-month fieldwork experience to allow students to develop entry-level skills in a specialty area, such as pediatrics, gerontology, or hand therapy. Direct supervision must be provided by a registered occupational therapist with at least one year of experience. For occupational therapy assistant students, direct supervision can be provided by an OTR or a COTA, also with a minimum of one year of experience. Ultimate responsibility for the Level II fieldwork experience must be assumed by a registered occupational therapist. Although the minimum requirement is one year of experience, fieldwork educators should be competent clinicians who can serve as good role models or mentors for our future practitioners.[2]

Occupational therapy students are expected to complete their fieldwork experience within 24 months following completion of academic preparation, while occupational therapy assistant students are expected to complete their Level II requirement within 12 months following completion of academic preparation. Some academic programs include the Level II fieldwork experiences in its degree requirements and offer corresponding academic credit, while other academic programs view the Level II fieldwork experience as a professional requirement and do not offer academic credit for the experience. In either case, successful completion of Level II fieldwork, or equivalent time, is an eligibility requirement for certification as a registered occupational therapist or assistant.

Roles and Responsibilities

While the emphasis of this chapter is developing a fieldwork program, we will first define the roles and responsibilities of each of the players involved in this collaborative endeavor.

Students

Occupational therapy students are eligible to begin their fieldwork experiences following successful completion of the appropriate academic coursework. For example, students should successfully complete the prerequisites for applying theory and practice to a psychosocial setting before beginning a fieldwork experience in such a setting. The decision-making process in choosing a fieldwork placement is viewed as an important step in students' education and career planning. Choosing a fieldwork placement is a collaborative multistage process in which academic fieldwork coordinators and the students review clinical interests, career goals, preferred clinical environments, financial needs, geographical concerns, learning style, personal strengths, and areas for growth. Synthesizing this information, students and coordinators identify potential fieldwork sites. Finally, the academic fieldwork coordinators negotiate the fieldwork arrangements with clinical sites.

Upon completion of the Level II fieldwork experience, students are expected to demonstrate competency in the areas of assessment, planning, treatment, problem solving, administration, and professionalism. The overall purpose of the fieldwork experience is to gain mastery in occupational therapy procedures and begin to develop the reasoning processes necessary for entry-level competence.

Although goals and objectives specific to each particular fieldwork setting will be individualized, students are expected to demonstrate competency in the administration and interpretation of evaluation procedures which are routinely utilized by occupational therapists in the given fieldwork setting. Based on the theoretical frame of reference practiced at the fieldwork setting, students should become proficient in implementing, justifying, and evaluating the effectiveness of their therapy with clients. Effective oral and written communication of ideas and objectives relevant to the roles and duties of an occupational therapist, including interactions with clients and staff in a professional manner are additional expectations of occupational therapy students. Moreover, students are responsible for demonstrating a sensitivity to and respect for client confidentiality. Finally, acquisition of professional characteristics that demonstrate the ability to establish and sustain therapeutic relationships and to work collaboratively with others will be expected in all fieldwork settings.[7]

The specific responsibilities of students are as follows:

- Fulfilling all duties and responsibilities identified by the fieldwork and academic fieldwork coordinators within the designated time frames.
- Complying with the professional standards identified by the fieldwork facility, the university, and the Principles of Occupational Therapy Code of Ethics as

revised by the Representative Assembly of the American Occupational Therapy Association in 1988 (refer to Figure 4-3).

- Communicating with fieldwork educators to confirm the starting dates and other prerequisite information.
- Securing documentation of adequate medical and professional insurance coverage for the duration of the fieldwork experience.
- Completing and presenting to the fieldwork educators one copy of students' evaluation of the fieldwork experience.[8]

Academic Fieldwork Coordinators

In each academic program an academic fieldwork coordinator functions as a liaison among the academic setting, the fieldwork center, and the students. The responsibilities of the academic fieldwork coordinator are outlined as follows:

1. Assigning eligible students to fieldwork experiences and confirming the assignment in writing to each fieldwork coordinator.
2. Assuring that all written contracts or letters of agreement between the academic institution and the fieldwork education center are signed and periodically reviewed may include negotiation with lawyers.
3. Making regular and periodic contacts with each fieldwork education center where students are placed.
4. Maintaining a current information file on each fieldwork education center where students are placed.
5. Identifying new sites for fieldwork education.
6. Developing and implementing a policy for withdrawal of students from a fieldwork center.
7. Orienting students to the general purposes of the fieldwork experience and providing them with the necessary forms.
8. Reassigning students who do not complete original fieldwork assignments in accordance with academic institution's policies.
9. Developing fieldwork experience programs that provide the best opportunity for the implementation of theoretical concepts offered as part of the academic curriculum.
10. Maintaining a collaborative relationship with fieldwork education centers.
11. Sending necessary information and forms for each student to the fieldwork coordinator/educator.[2]

Knowledge of fieldwork education programs is an important aspect of the academic fieldwork coordinator's job to accurately represent the fieldwork programs to students. Accordingly, periodic visits are made to the fieldwork centers to review fieldwork program learning opportunities and expectations for students. When on-site visits are unrealistic, telephone communication is an alternative. The academic fieldwork coordinator is available for consultation to both students and fieldwork educators/coordinators and frequently serves as a mediator when problems arise. In this role the academic coordinator can serve as an objective third person to help students and fieldwork educators identify concerns and develop a mutually acceptable plan of action.

Fieldwork Coordinators and Educators

Fieldwork educators assume responsibility for the direct day-to-day supervision of students. These individuals must be occupational therapists, registered with a minimum of one year of experience in direct client services. Although *fieldwork educator* is the official AOTA title for the direct supervisor's role, *clinical educator, fieldwork supervisor* or *student supervisor* are all interchangeable titles.[2] In large occupational therapy departments coordination and administration of the fieldwork program might be delegated to one staff person with specific requirements written into the job description. This person is commonly called the *fieldwork coordinator* and assumes responsibility for the management of the entire fieldwork program including negotiating with the academic fieldwork coordinators, scheduling students, designing and evaluating the fieldwork program, training and supervising the fieldwork educators' direct supervision of students, and functioning as a facilitator for students' growth and development. The staff member appointed as the fieldwork coordinator should be proficient as a clinician, experienced in clinical education, interested in students, possess good interpersonal relationship and organizational skills, and be knowledgeable of the facility and its resources. If the clinical facility trains two or more students at a time, on a year-round basis, fieldwork coordination will take up from 25 to 50% of a staff person's time. Therefore, the fieldwork coordinator should only be expected to function at a 50 to 75% treatment productivity level as compared to other full-time staff members.[10]

The fieldwork educator, as differentiated from the coordinator, should also be interested and willing to work with students, proficient as a clinician, enthusiastic, sensitive to students, receptive to feedback, and possess strong interpersonal skills. During the fieldwork experience, fieldwork educators initially spend much time with students, which decreases the clinician's ability to provide direct treatment; however, research indicates that students add to productivity later in the fieldwork experience.[4,6,16,17] Therefore, it is appropriate to expect that the fieldwork educator will only be able to function at 50 to 75% productivity during the first few weeks of the fieldwork experience, returning to higher levels of productivity as demands for supervision decrease. When the fieldwork educator is expected to perform at optimal productivity and supervise a student, unsatisfactory experiences result, often leading to burnout. Large occupational therapy departments often have one fieldwork coordinator and many fieldwork educators. In smaller occupational therapy departments, one person can assume responsibility for both of these roles.

The job of the fieldwork coordinator can be characterized as having two primary components. On the one hand are the administrative responsibilities of the fieldwork coordinator, which include, but are not limited to, the following:

- Collaborating with the academic fieldwork coordinator in the development of a fieldwork program that provides the best opportunity for the implementation of theoretical concepts offered as part of the academic program;

- Creating an environment that facilitates learning, clinical inquiry and reflection upon one's practice;
- Preparing, maintaining, and sending to the academic fieldwork coordinator current information about the fieldwork center, including a statement of the conceptual models from which evaluation is derived, and upon which therapy is based;
- Scheduling students in collaboration with the academic fieldwork coordinator;
- Identifying the philosophy of the fieldwork center and establishing objectives of the fieldwork experience;
- Overseeing the direct supervision of students by meeting regularly with fieldwork educators and contributing to the evaluation of each student at midpoint and upon completion of the fieldwork experience;
- Being familiar with the policy regarding the "withdrawal of students from fieldwork experience" of each academic institution from which students are accepted; and notifying the academic fieldwork coordinator of any student for whom the fieldwork center is requesting withdrawal or other problems that can arise;
- Reviewing periodically the contractual agreement between the academic institution and the fieldwork education center and ensuring that these agreements are signed by the appropriate parties before students begin the fieldwork experience. This might include consultation with the clinical facilities' lawyers.

Administrative duties are supplemented by the direct day-to-day supervisory responsibilities of the fieldwork educator, which include, but are not limited to:

- Providing an adequate orientation to the fieldwork education center and to specific department policies and procedures;
- Assigning patients to students, defining expectations clearly to students;
- Supervising the provision of occupational therapy services; documentation and oral reporting of students;
- Assessing skills, knowledge, and attitudes of students;
- Meeting with students regularly to review performance and to provide guidance and feedback that uses behavioral language and observable data. As a result of the fieldwork educator's feedback, goals for change are developed collaboratively between students and fieldwork educators;
- Seeking evaluation of one's own supervisory skills from appropriate people.[2]

Designing the Fieldwork Program

The creation of a fieldwork education program results from the integration of a facility's purpose and objectives, the academic program, the occupational therapy department itself, and our beliefs about education in the situation of practice. The fieldwork education center should be prepared to meet the minimum requirements of an approved fieldwork education center established in the *Essentials and Guidelines of an Accredited Educational Program for the Occupational Therapist and Occupational Therapy Assistant*. These include the following:

- Fieldwork education centers shall be approved by recognized accrediting agencies or meet standards established by the academic program.
- Fieldwork shall be conducted in settings approved by the educational program as providing experiences appropriate to the learning needs of the students and as meeting objectives of fieldwork.
- The ratio of fieldwork supervisors to students shall be such as to ensure quality experience and maximal learning.
- Level I fieldwork shall be supervised by qualified personnel.
- Level II fieldwork for the occupational therapy student shall be supervised by a registered occupational therapist; the Level II occupational therapy assistant student's fieldwork experience shall be the responsibility of a registered occupational therapist, with supervision provided by an OTR or COTA. Supervising OTRs and COTAs shall have a minimum of one year of experience.[2]

In preparation for designing a fieldwork program, the fieldwork coordinator, department director, or person responsible for designing the fieldwork program first needs to identify and analyze many of the variables that will influence the fieldwork program. As noted earlier, the clinical facility, occupational therapy department, occupational therapy academic programs, and educational beliefs will all affect the design and structure of the entire fieldwork program. For example, the fieldwork program in a pediatric rehabilitation teaching facility in which a large occupational therapy department provides services for learning disabled children will obviously differ significantly from the fieldwork program in an acute care hospital, with a three-person department. Once these variables have been carefully analyzed, the fieldwork coordinator can decide whether or not a fieldwork educational program is a realistic endeavor for the occupational therapy department to pursue. Careful analysis of the complex systems will provide the foundation for making the decision and, if the fieldwork coordinator chooses to proceed, implementing a fieldwork program. As an analysis of the various systems will serve as the basis for the fieldwork program design, we will first examine the clinical facility (Figure 8-1).

Clinical Facility

Every organization is designed to achieve certain goals. Providing social or human services to individuals is the most likely primary goal of facilities in which occupational therapists work. In some facilities, teaching and research are secondary goals that are clearly

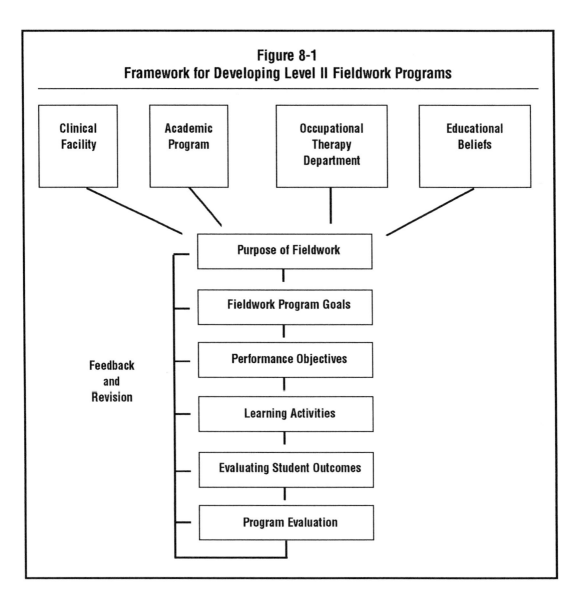

Figure 8-1
Framework for Developing Level II Fieldwork Programs

stated in the facility's mission statement, while in other settings teaching is not an organizational priority. In either case, the fieldwork coordinator needs to be cognizant of the facilities' primary goals and assess how and where the goal of preparing future practitioners intersects with those of the organization. Answers to the following questions will influence the fieldwork coordinator's decision:

- Facility Goals: Does administration support fieldwork education? If so, what kind of support? (Verbal support, space, allocation of staff to design program, funding for stipends or educational materials such as books, etc.?). If not, is there potential to gain support?
- Funding Source: How is the organization funded? Will the funding source have an impact on the fieldwork program?

- Referral Source: What is the referral mechanism? Will there be a constant client population for fieldwork students to treat? What kind of pressures does the referral mechanism create for supervisors?
- Types of Clients and Length of Stay: Who does the facility provide services for, when, and for how long are the clients available? Are there an adequate variety and number of clients available for students to treat?
- Facility Staff and Patterns: Who are the other members of the service delivery team? Is the staffing consistent? Do other members of the team offer fieldwork education? Is there access to interdisciplinary education such as rounds, case conferences, or inservices?
- Support Services: What kind of support services are available to students? Examples of possible support services might include: health care, emergency medical care, library facilities, meals, housing, duplicating or computer services, parking, or even stipends?
- Accreditation: Does the facility meet current accreditation (JCAH, CARF, state licensing) standards? Does the facility provide safe and healthy working conditions?

Occupational Therapy Department

The philosophy and structure of the occupational therapy department itself will have the most significant impact on the design of the fieldwork program. Decisions such as the structure of supervisory responsibilities, the number of schools you will accept students from, how you communicate with the schools, how often you will accept students, the types of educational experiences offered, and the student expectations are all dependent upon a thorough analysis of the occupational therapy department. The following questions can serve as a guide for analyzing the occupational therapy department component of the entire system.

- Occupational Therapy Department Frame of Reference: Are occupational therapy services provided within the context of a specific framework and how does it affect the provision of occupational therapy services?
- Scope of Occupational Therapy Services: What domains of functioning does occupational therapy address? What kinds of experiences will students be exposed to? Are there opportunities available for a range of experiences in screening, evaluation, planning, treatment implementation, reevaluation, follow up, and reporting? Are there specialized programs within the occupational therapy department? If so, do therapists need advanced skills or can these programs be implemented by entry-level therapists?
- Occupational Therapy Staffing Patterns: What is the current staffing pattern? Is there a consistent staff available to supervise students? What is the expectation of

the facility administration? Is the fieldwork program viewed as a mechanism to strengthen the quality of services by ensuring that staff keep abreast of current theory and practice? Is the fieldwork program viewed as a viable means of recruitment?

- Space and Equipment: What kind of space is available for extra people? Is there room in the clinic for another person? Is there enough equipment available for planned learning experiences? Is there room in the department to set aside an appropriate work and writing space for students? Is there a place to store educationally related materials that are accessible to students? Is there a private area for counseling students and providing private feedback?
- Client Schedules: Are client schedules conducive to students' schedules? If necessary, is it possible to fit additional treatment sessions into the client's schedule?
- Potential Costs and Benefits of Fieldwork Program: Some of the potential benefits of a fieldwork program are expanded staff recruitment possibilities, promotion of continuing education opportunities for staff personnel through liaison with academic institutions such as workshops, access to libraries, tuition remission and the challenge of keeping abreast of current theories and practice, public relations for the clinical facility and availability of additional personnel to provide client services. Most of the costs are incurred in staff supervision and planning time. Do the benefits offset the costs to your facility?

Academic Program

Once the analysis of the clinical facility and the occupational therapy department are completed, we turn our attention to the academic programs. Initially it is important to consider whether the academic program and clinical facility's philosophies, objectives for client care, and expectations for fieldwork education are compatible. Because students are placed in fieldwork settings to apply and practice theory and techniques taught in the academic setting, the clinical facility should be aware of the academic program's philosophical orientation, curricula, and fieldwork requirements. Likewise, the academic program should be aware of the learning experiences available in the clinical setting. Each academic program will delineate general fieldwork objectives that are consistent with the knowledge and skills utilized at the fieldwork facilities. It is the clinic's responsibility to then delineate the learning objectives specific to their setting.

During initial contacts with academic fieldwork coordinators, it is advisable to reach a mutual understanding of communication expectations and scheduling mechanisms. Pedantic as they might seem, issues such as who will receive the communication or when the academic program schedules placements will be crucial to the success of the fieldwork program. Grounds for termination of a student's fieldwork, how termination should be documented, and what are the withdrawal and retention policies of the school are examples of the many issues that need to be negotiated between academic institutions and fieldwork facilities. The result of these negotiations is the preparation of a memorandum of understanding between the two facilities.

Academic programs and clinical facilities sign a legal contract that outline the areas of responsibility between the two institutions. Because legal consequences can often be serious, as well as costly, the occupational therapy administrator is urged to consult competent counsel whenever an apparent legal issue arises. The contracts that are reviewed by lawyers representing the two institutions usually cover the following components:

- Specification of duties and obligations, rights and responsibilities of clinical facility, academic institution and student
- Health status of student and required health tests
- Limits of personal and professional liability insurance
- Procedural and enforcement of provisions, grievance, dismissal of student, and termination of agreement
- If applicable, financial provisions (stipends, room, board)
- Renewal provisions

Because all fieldwork placements are contingent upon the signing of this contractual agreement by clinical facilities and academic programs, students might not begin their fieldwork placements until the contracts are acceptable and signed. Once the terms of the contracts are negotiated and signed by both parties, a copy is filed at each setting for reference.

Educational Belief

Each occupational therapy department identifies a conceptual frame of reference that defines the domains of service provided by the department. Similarly, each occupational therapy department must identify its underlying beliefs about education and learning that will be reflected in its approach to fieldwork. Since it is only possible here to select a few examples of the perspectives that seem to be congruent with the field of occupational therapy, fieldwork coordinators might benefit from reviewing various educational perspectives and identifying what effect their beliefs will have on the design of the fieldwork program.

Particularly relevant to occupational therapy fieldwork education is the work of Jerome Brunner. He stresses the importance of learning a basic idea that can be used for recognizing subsequent problems as special cases of the original idea, which is continually broadened and deepened. He claims that a "grasping a general idea makes it available for subsequent phenomena."[3] Therefore, unless detail is placed in a structured framework, it is rapidly forgotten. Learning a skill without understanding the underlying concepts and principles limits the transference of knowledge from one situation to another. The fieldwork educator who finds Brunner's perspective useful to fieldwork education can then structure the fieldwork experience to ensure that students understand underlying concepts such as normal range of movement before they apply the concept to a variety of clients.

Philosopher John Dewey's writing also provides occupational therapists with a useful perspective on fieldwork education. One of the many ideas Dewey advocates is individualized education. He claims education must be phrased in the language of the learner:

> Teaching carries with it the responsibility for understanding the needs and capacities of the individuals who are learning at a given time. It is not enough that certain material and methods have proved effective with other individuals at other times. It is important to pay attention to what is educative with particular individuals at particular times.[11]

Fieldwork educators, unlike academic educators, have the luxury of a one-to-one relationship with each student. The relationship allows the fieldwork educator to consider the individual needs of the learner in order to custom-design the learning experience within the context of the clinical setting. The educator might then wish to spend some time initially assessing students' particular learning needs and developing mutually agreed upon objectives within the context of the entry-level expectations outlined by the fieldwork educator. Opportunities for discussion of and feedback about students' strengths and areas for growth can be scheduled on an ongoing basis to facilitate individualized learning.

As occupational therapy students emerge from the role of students to the professional role of clinicians, they will need to develop independence in pursuing and integrating the knowledge associated with learning tasks. They must surrender the student role in which they are dependent upon faculty to determine the content of their learning and begin to take responsibility for their own professional growth. Malcome Knowles, the seminal figure in the field of adult education, highlights the usefulness of learning theories and educational approaches for adults that foster a climate characterized by increased motivation to learn, critical inquiry, and individualization of the learning experience. Knowles stresses the value of building the learning experience upon the prior knowledge and life experience of the learner. His perspective blends well with Dewey's ideas of custom-designing the learning experience. Adult learners enter a learning situation with a rich array of past experiences and previous learning. Knowles claims that adult learners know their learning style and can identify the circumstances in which they are most successful as learners.[13] To custom-design the learning experience to accommodate students' past experiences and learning styles, many fieldwork educators have designed learning style inventories and questionnaires to invite students to share their personalized learning style and assess their past experience in relation to the expectations of the fieldwork setting. Table 8-1 provides an example in which students are asked to identify their past experience with particular evaluation tools and treatment methodologies.

These questionnaires might also alleviate unnecessary work for fieldwork educators. If fieldwork educators initially take the time to assess what students need to learn they might avoid duplication of previous learning and negation of students' prior knowledge and skill.

Other forms of identifying students' readiness to perform a given clinical task with actual clients include observation of students performing a similar task, simulating the situation or asking students for self-assessments of their readiness. All of these strategies constitute ways in which the fieldwork educator determines whether or not students are ready to function at the level of knowledge, independence, or judgment required for the task. Furthermore, these strategies provide mechanisms for the fieldwork educators to minimize the risks involved in ensuring the welfare of clients. The concern for clients is the top priority and influences all fieldwork education activities. Since client care can occasionally conflict with educational goals for students, the fieldwork education experiences must be structured to support the professional ethos of providing the quality care for clients at all times.

The adult learner is motivated to achieve when the learning is immediately applied. It isn't enough that the fieldwork educator feels that a particular learning activity is important, it must be perceived as important by students as well. One underlying component of successful learning experience for the adult is the communication expectations. Expectations must be known before they can be met. Therefore, fieldwork educators might want to share their expectations and rationale for designing a particular learning experience so students understand why they are being asked to engage in a particular activity. Together students and fieldwork educators might then identify the specific skills to be learned and resulting learning activities for the fieldwork experience.

These are just a few examples of educational beliefs that can impact the design of the fieldwork program. The fieldwork coordinator might further explore educational beliefs by asking members of the occupational therapy department to answer questions such as: What do we believe about the learning process? How do people learn? What facilitates learning? What does it mean to learn? How will we know when learning has taken place? What do we believe about learning in occupational therapy? If answers to such questions are defined, the fieldwork program can be designed and evaluated against these identified beliefs.

Purpose of Fieldwork Program

Once the clinical facility, academic program, occupational therapy department, and educational beliefs are analyzed, the fieldwork coordinator is ready to utilize the analysis to explicate the purpose of the fieldwork program in the given clinical facility. Although the overall purpose of the fieldwork experience is to provide occupational therapy students with the opportunity to integrate academic knowledge with application skills to develop competency as entry-level therapists or assistants, each clinical facility will need to identify the unique aspects of its program. It is expected that students will gain knowledge and refine skills consistent with those utilized at the fieldwork centers. For example, a therapist working in a children's hospital might decide that the purpose of the fieldwork program is to prepare clinicians to work in pediatric settings only, while a therapist working in a large rehabilitation hospital might decide to design a fieldwork program that offers students a generic preparation for working in a variety of settings.

Table 8-1
Occupational Therapy Department
Student Questionnaire

The following questionnaire is to be filled out at the onset of your affiliation in order to help the occupational therapy staff plan a meaningful experience for you.

Name: **Date:**

Expectations:
What is your understanding of this facility, i.e., types of clientele we serve?

What are your expectations of this affiliation and what are the skills you wish to leave with? Identify special areas of interest in O.T.

Functioning of Self Strengths:
Identify strong skills that you know will maximize your learning potential.

Weaknesses:
Identify those qualities that you would like to improve upon, which you feel could be realistically achieved upon completion of this affiliation.

Table 8-1 (continued)

Learning Style
Source of Motivation:
Do you prefer to have goals set and motivation supplied by
a. _____ supervisor's expectations and directions
b. _____ expectations of schools
c. _____ your own personal expectations and interests
d. _____ combination of a and c

Supervision for New Tasks:
When learning a new task, do you prefer
a. _____ observing demonstration of task with discussion following?
b. _____ completing task on your own, demonstrating the task with discussion following?
c. _____ discussion before and after task?

Approach to Content:
When learning something new do you usually prefer
a. _____ to find out the rationale for it first, understand the whole process and then start to work on practical specifics?
b. _____ to get right into practical aspects at the beginning and wait to learn theory after you have gotten a chance to practice the specifics?

Need for Feedback:
How frequently do you seem to need feedback on how you are doing during learning?
a. _____ several times initially and infrequently after that
b. _____ fairly frequently until you have made substantial progress in mastery, then infrequently
c. _____ frequently even after you seem to have mastered the skill

Type of Feedback:
What type(s) of feedback seem to be most helpful?
a. _____ praise from instructor or other expert
b. _____ approval of peers, other staff members
c. _____ being told your performance is correct or incorrect and why
d. _____ seeing practical results you believe are related to your performance
e. _____ receiving guidelines and criteria beforehand and then receiving feedback on the identified criteria

Table 8-1 (continued)

Please check off your understanding of the following formal and informal evaluations and treatment techniques.

Standardized tests	Don't know	Have observed others administer test	Help needed	Can administer
Gessell Developmental Scale				
Beery Test of Visual Motor Integration				
Frostig Developmental Test of Visual Perception				
McCarthy Scales of Children's Abilities				
Raven Progressive Matrices				
Knox Cubes Test				
SCSIT—Visual Porcoption Toct				
SCSIT—Motor Accuracy				
SCSIT—Right/Left Discrimination				
MacQuarrie Test of Mechanical Ability				
Minnesota Rate of Manipulation Test				
Motor Free Visual Perception Test				
Detroit Memory for Designs				
Evaluations				
Developmental Assessments				
Prevocational Assessments				
Reflex Testing				
Range of Motion				
Muscle Testing				
Feeding				
Nonvocal Communication				
Sensation				
Coordination—Gross & Fine				
Dressing				
Grooming/Hygiene				
Home Assessments				

Table 8-1 (continued)

Standardized tests	Don't know	Have observed others administer test	Help needed	Can administer
Multisensory Treatment Approach				
Positioning and Handling				
Wheelchair Positioning				
Splint Construction				
Adaptive Equipment (what kind)				
Feeding				
Dressing				
Training in Fine Motor Activities				
Training in Math/Problem Solving				
Range of Motion and Muscle Reeducation				
Behavior Management				
Gross Motor				
Sensory Integration				
Sensory Stimulation				
Socialization				
Functional Skill Development				
Family Teaching				
Hygiene				
Prevocational				
Communication				

In order to plan your learning experiences to fit your individual special interests and career goals, please check the following:

Age Levels	Extremely Interested	Moderately Interested	Not Interested
$3^1/_2$-5			
5-8			
8-13			
13-21			

Special Interests—rate areas 1-8 with #1 being most interested

Sensory integration		Prevocational training	
Feeding		Dressing	
Nonvocal communication		Creative technological aids	
Math training		Research	

Performance Objectives and Learning Activities

Prepared with the information from the above analysis, including a notion of the overall purpose of the fieldwork program, the fieldwork coordinator can use the objective setting process to identify the specific learning experiences and expectations for students. Objectives accomplish many things in the design and structure of the fieldwork program, but the most important reason for objectives is to clearly delineate performance expectations for students. The process of writing exactly what you expect students to be able to do when they complete their fieldwork forces the fieldwork coordinator to identify what learning experiences to offer. Organizationally, the objectives can be used as a means for planning the learning experiences for students. The objectives also serve as a guide to evaluate students' performance. Since the AOTA Fieldwork Evaluation for the Occupational Therapist or the AOTA Fieldwork Evaluation Form for Occupational Therapy Assistant Students are the formally recognized tools utilized to evaluate students' entry-level performance upon completion of the fieldwork experience, it is recommended that the fieldwork coordinator develop performance objectives and learning experiences that reflect the items addressed on these evaluation forms. For example, the Occupational Therapy Assistant Evaluation Form addresses the student's ability to communicate with relevant others to facilitate collaborative implementation of overall treatment goals. Thus, students should have the opportunity to interact with others in planning treatment goals. The learning activity becomes either the treatment team planning meeting or the student might seek out relevant others on an individualized basis. In this example, we see that the learning activities directly result from the defined performance objectives.

Writing Performance Objectives

Prior to the student's arrival, the fieldwork coordinator will need to define the entry-level competencies, written in the form of performance objectives. These performance objectives describe the entry-level competencies necessary for safe and effective practice within the given clinical facility.

An objective is an intent communicated by a statement describing what the student should know or demonstrate that he or she is able to do as a result of the learning experience. Objectives should describe just what the instructor or evaluator should be able to observe in the student's performance when the objective has been reached. "An objective is a description of a performance you want learners to be able to exhibit before you consider them competent."[14] In all of these definitions, the focus is on the action performed by students. Therefore, objectives with action verbs state what students must do to show achievement.

Criteria for a well-written behavioral objective include three essential components:

1. *Performance:* observable behavior of student
   Statement describes what learner will be doing (learner activity) when he or she is demonstrating that he or she has reached the objective.
2. *Condition:* specifics of a situation

Statement describes the important conditions (givens and other restrictions) under which the learner will be expected to demonstrate his or her competence.

3. *Criteria:* acceptable level of performance in measurable terms (speed, quality, degree of achievement)

   Statement indicates how the learner will be evaluated and the acceptable performance.

The following example is an objective written to correspond to the AOTA Fieldwork Education for the Occupational Therapist. Since students' performance will be evaluated by this evaluation tool, the performance objective defines the condition and criteria for the evaluation item number 46, "Participates responsibly in the supervisory relationship."[9]

"Given weekly one hour supervisory sessions, the student will responsibly participate in supervisory sessions by attending all scheduled supervision meetings prepared, submitting verbal and written material in a prompt manner, initiating agenda items to be discussed in supervision and changing behavior in response to supervisory feedback."

The condition is described as one hour weekly supervision, the performance states that the student will participate and the criteria includes the acceptable levels of performance. Stating requirements to be prepared, prompt, acting with initiative, and changing in response to supervision all describe the expected outcomes.

Although initially quite time consuming, it is well worth the fieldwork coordinators' and educators' efforts to clearly delineate the performance expectations and measurement criteria before they are confronted with the formal evaluation of students. This evaluation requires the student and fieldwork educator to assess learner performance in achieving the objective. This feedback is essential for the students' development. Each student and fieldwork educator must determine how effectively the learning experience has provided the student with the knowledge, skills, and attitude to demonstrate achievement of the performance objective. All evaluation of clinical performance involves differences of interpretation and is, therefore, subjective to some extent. Performance objectives minimize the subjectivity and provide fieldwork educators with a mechanism to fairly evaluate each student with the same criteria.

Student and Program Evaluation

Once the performance objectives, resulting learning activities, and student outcomes are determined, the fieldwork coordinator will need to assess the efficacy of the overall fieldwork program. Since the overall purpose of the fieldwork program is to provide students with the opportunities necessary to develop entry-level competencies, the evaluation must first look at students' performance results and then at the design of the entire program. The first factor is dependent upon individual student variables and the second, program factor, is dependent upon the design and structure of the educational experience provided. Formative and summative evaluations are necessary to accomplish the goals of both student and program evaluation.

Formative evaluation takes place while the fieldwork program is ongoing to help students determine their progress toward the expected competencies, strengths, areas of growth, and plans for the remainder of the fieldwork experience. AOTA recommends utilizing the standard evaluation forms (Fieldwork Evaluation for Therapists or Fieldwork Evaluation for Assistants) at the midpoint of the fieldwork experience for these formative purposes of evaluating students' performance.

To assess the fieldwork program structure, many fieldwork centers design their own feedback forms. Common items on such forms include questions about the orientation to the facility, the assignments and treatment caseload, structure of the fieldwork program, supervision, and communication. These forms provide students and fieldwork educators with a springboard to discuss their impressions of the experience to date and make necessary changes while time allows. Formative evaluation does not need to be limited to formalized supervision meetings with standardized forms. This type of ongoing evaluation might likewise occur informally after a therapy session or at the end of the day. Fieldwork educators and students will benefit from carefully monitoring the learning experience.

Summative evaluation, on the other hand, determines how well the final goals were actually met at the end of the program. The AOTA standardized forms are utilized to assess students' performance upon completion of the fieldwork experience. These forms are the formally recognized tools for evaluation because they serve as a mechanism for monitoring who enters our profession. All students must successfully complete their fieldwork experiences to be eligible for the national certification examination. Presently, the Student Evaluation of Fieldwork Experience (SEFWE) is the instrument for use by occupational therapy and occupational therapy assistant students to assess the fieldwork experience itself. The SEFWE provides a mechanism for students to contribute "directly to the process of the fieldwork program development by documenting his or her perception of the program and suggesting changes."[2]

The problem is not so much finding information to evaluate as deciding what information is necessary to supplement these standardized tests. To avoid being inundated, you will need to limit the data gathering to answer specific questions such as, "Why did a particular student have difficulty with formulating treatment goals for a client with a right hemiparesis?"

The evaluation process begins by assessing the student's knowledge base. If the student has a solid understanding of the client diagnosis and is able to demonstrate an understanding of the treatment planning process, the fieldwork educator might need to assess the design of the fieldwork program. The fieldwork program should provide the student with opportunities to learn the entry-level competencies. Therefore, the fieldwork educator will need to assess whether the program has met the student's learning needs. Even though a student has observed a therapist provide therapy for clients, perhaps the student needs to observe another therapist provide therapy for a client with similar diagnosis. This observation might be followed with a discussion of the therapists' reasoning about the therapy plan. This type of formative evaluation can be utilized to facilitate the learning experience and help both students and fieldwork educators determine the most suitable learning experiences for a given student. The fieldwork educator can then use this information to revise the fieldwork program. Revision of content, organization, and approach is a constant process based on the findings of evaluations, learning and results.

Summary

The fieldwork experience plays an integral role in our professional preparation. Efficacious fieldwork education programs rely on an interdependent relationship between the key players. Therefore, it is essential that academic and clinical fieldwork coordinators develop collaborative relationships to design fieldwork education programs. The design of the fieldwork program is based upon a systemic analysis of the clinical facility, the occupational therapy department, the academic programs, and the educational beliefs of the occupational therapy department. Once careful analysis of these variables is completed, the clinical fieldwork coordinator develops learning experiences that consider the needs of the learner and teach the necessary entry-level competencies for the occupational therapy profession. The entire fieldwork program, including student performance, is evaluated on both a formative and summative basis.

Questions

1. The purpose of the Level II fieldwork experience is to:
   a. Duplicate academic education
   b. Promote clinical reasoning and reflective practice
   c. Allow students to observe clinical practice

2. Choosing a fieldwork placement is a collaborative process in which academic fieldwork coordinators and students identify potential fieldwork sites for students. Which of the following is not a critical factor in this decision making process?
   a. Weather
   b. Clinical interests
   c. Financial needs

3. In a large occupational therapy department, who is responsible for the direct day-to-day supervision of students?
   a. Academic fieldwork coordinator
   b. Fieldwork educator
   c. Fieldwork coordinator

4. The design of the fieldwork program is based on:
   a. The goals of the academic program and the fieldwork educator
   b. AOTA guidelines
   c. The integration of a facility's purpose and objectives, the academic program, the occupational therapy department, and our beliefs about education in the situation of practice

5. In designing a fieldwork program, the administrator first needs to:
   a. Establish performance objectives
   b. Analyze the systems, including the clinical facility and occupational therapy department, to determine the viability of developing a program
   c. Assess student's needs

6. Structuring the fieldwork experience to ensure that students understand underlying concepts is based on the notion that:
   a. Learning should be phrased in the language of the learner
   b. Learning a basic idea helps students recognize subsequent problems as special cases of the original idea
   c. Learning should consider one's past experience

7. The most important reasons for developing specific objectives is to:
   a. Document program requirements for academic fieldwork coordinators
   b. Meet AOTA guidelines
   c. Clearly delineate performance expectations for students

8. Identify the three essential components of a behavioral objective.
    a. Skills, actions, and goals
    b. Performance, judgment, and attitude
    c. Performance, condition, and criteria

9. Formative evaluation takes place:
    a. On the first day of the fieldwork experience
    b. At the midterm
    c. Both of the above

10. Summative evaluation:
    a. Determines how well the final goals were met at the end of the program
    b. Is ongoing
    c. Is used at midterm

Answers
1. b
2. a
3. b
4. c
5. b
6. b
7. c
8. c
9. c
10. a

Case Study 1

The director of the occupational therapy department at a state facility for adults with developmental disabilities asks you to develop a fieldwork program for occupational therapy students. The department is comprised of 20 occupational therapists who provide services for 500 adults in 4 different divisions within the facility. To determine the viability of establishing a fieldwork program, you begin by analyzing the clinical facility.

The first step is to meet with a representative from the facility administration. Since the facility presently provides training for other professional students, the administration recognizes the professional and financial benefits of such programs. Moreover, the training programs have served as an excellent recruitment source for the facility. Because of the tremendous revenue saved by avoiding advertising costs and recruitment time, the administration is willing to offer a small stipend to students. The administration would be delighted to support the occupational therapy department's fieldwork program.

The facility is publicly funded by the state department of mental health, therefore, therapists do not have to charge clients for individual therapy units. This allows the therapists flexibility to design therapy programs that will in turn allow you to develop a flexible fieldwork program.

Because the facility provides residential care for adults with chronic needs, there is a constant and stable patient population. You determine that you will have the luxury to tailor design the student's caseload because you will know what client population will be available at a given time. In analyzing the client population from an educational perspective, you realize that there is a tremendous variety in the clinical needs, creating potentially variable learning experiences. Examples of the domains of services provided by the occupational therapy department include: positioning and wheelchair adaptations, neurodevelopmental treatment, sensory-motor treatment, mealtime programs, activity of daily living programs, vocational programs, consultation to day programs and workshops, annual evaluations, and consultation to direct-care staff. Because the clinical needs are developmental, psychological, and physical, you make the decision to design a fieldwork program for students who have completed fieldwork experiences in settings that provide services addressing both psychosocial and physical dysfunction needs. Furthermore, your program will be marketed to the academic programs as a specialty experience for students who have an interest in developmental disabilities.

As you continue your analysis of the clinical facility, you learn that there is an interdisciplinary seminar for psychology, social work, physical therapy, and speech therapy students. The seminar is led by a developmental psychologist and addresses current issues in the care and delivery services for developmental disabled adults. Topics such as transition to community placements, philosophies of workshop settings, or use of behavioral interventions are discussed. The psychologist would be delighted to have occupational therapy students participate in the seminar. This confirms your decision to market the fieldwork experience as a specialty experience in developmental disabilities. As you complete the analysis of the clinical facility you then call the academic fieldwork coordinator at the local occupational therapy schools to determine their needs and assess whether or not your program will match their needs.

Case Study 2

The AOTA Fieldwork Evaluation for the Occupational Therapist addresses students' ability to administer assessment procedures according to standardized techniques. Since students' performance will be evaluated by this evaluation tool, the fieldwork coordinator determined that students will need to learn to administer the standardized test used at the clinical facility. The fieldwork coordinator writes a behavioral objective delineating the performance expectations and measurement criteria.

You, the fieldwork educator, agree with Dewey's notion that education should be individualized and phrased in the language of the learner. Likewise, you believe Knowles' ascertainment that the adult learners know their learning style and can identify successful learning situations. Finally, you are committed to the philosophy that the supervisory relationship is a collaborative process in which both fieldwork educators and students are responsible for planning learning experiences.

Based on these beliefs you decide to ask the student how she would like to approach learning the standardized evaluations. Together you and the student determine that the student would like to first read the test manual and then observe someone administer the test. After the observation the student will practice administering the test with another student. Finally, the student will administer the test to you. You will provide feedback before the student administers the test to a client. This collaborative approach to designing learning experiences is then used throughout the fieldwork program.

References

1. American Occupational Therapy Association. *Essentials and Guidelines of an Accredited Educational Program for the Occupational Therapist.* 1991.
2. American Occupational Therapy Association. *Guide to Fieldwork Education.* Rockville, MD: American Occupational Therapy Association, 1985.
3. Bruner J. *The Process of Education.* New York: Vintage Books, 1963.
4. Burkhardt BF. A time study of staff and student activities in a level II fieldwork program. *Am J Occup Ther.* 39:35-40, 1985.
5. Christie B, Joyce P, Moeller P. Fieldwork experience, part 1: Impact on practice preference. *Am J Occup Ther.* 37:817-823, 1983.
6. Chung YI, Spelbring LM. An analysis of weekly instructional input hours and student work hours in occupational therapy fieldwork. *Am J Occup Ther.* 37:681-687, 1983.
7. Cohn E. Fieldwork Education: Applying Theory to Practice. In HL Hopkins and HD Smith (eds): *Willard and Spackman's Occupational Therapy.* 7th ed. Philadelphia: J.B. Lippincott, 1988.
8. Cohn E. *Student Fieldwork Manual.* Medford, MA: Tufts University-Boston School of Occupational Therapy, 1986.
9. Commission on Education of the American Occupational Therapy Association. *Fieldwork Evaluation for the Occupational Therapist.* Rockville, MD: American Occupational Therapy Association, 1986.
10. Curtis K. *Organizing and Facilitating a Clinical Education Program: A Course for the Clinical Coordinator.* 2nd ed. Los Angeles: Health Directions, 1986.
11. Dewey J. *Experience and Education.* New York: MacMillan, 1938.

12. Fidler G. Learning as a growth process: A conceptual framework for professional education. *Am J Occup Ther.* 20:1-8, 1966.

13. Knowles M. *The Modern Practice of Adult Education.* New York: Association Press, 1980.

14. Mager R. *Preparing Instructional Objectives.* 2nd ed. California: Fearon Publishers, 1975.

15. Nystrom E. The differentiation between academic and fieldwork education. *Occupational Therapy Education: Target 2000 Proceedings.* Rockville, MD: American Occupational Therapy Association, 1986.

16. Page GG, MacKinnor JR. Cost of clinical instructors' time in clinical education—Physical therapy students. *Phys Ther.* 67:238-243, 1987.

17. Shalik LD. Cost-benefit analysis of level II fieldwork in occupational therapy. *Am J Occup Ther.* 41:638-645, 1987.

Suggested Readings

1. American Physical Therapy Association. *Standards for Clinical Education in Physical Therapy—A Manual for Evaluation and Selection of Clinical Education Centers.* Alexandria, VA: American Physical Therapy Association, 1981.

2. Cohn ES. Fieldwork education: Shaping a foundation for clinical reasoning. *Am J Occup Ther.* 43:240-244, 1989.

3. Crepeau EB, Lagarde T. (Eds.) *Clinical Education and Supervision: An Instructional Guide.* Rockville, MD: American Occupational Therapy Association, 1991.

4. Crist P. *Contemporary Issues in Clinical Education.* Thorofare, NJ: SLACK, 1986.

CHAPTER 9

Quality Management in Occupational Therapy

Martha K. Logigian, MS, OTR/L
Laurel Cargill Radley, MS, OTR

Introduction

Quality management (QM) in health care is the systematic effort to determine if care is provided at an acceptable level. It reflects the degree of adherence to standards of good practice and achievement of anticipated outcome. A common approach to assessing quality care has been to establish a program which measures performance to assure that it conforms to pre-established standards, i.e., decrease variation of a process. In cases where performance fails to conform, providers attempt to improve behavior via change of intervention or improvement in technique or skill.

History

The concept of quality management began in England in the nineteenth century. In the United States a means of health care assessment was developed using case histories and re-evaluation of patients one year after discharge to determine whether care had been satisfactory. At the same time, the recognition of the unacceptable conditions of hospitals made the medical community cognizant of the need for improvement. In 1918, the American College of Surgeons established a voluntary accreditation process which set minimum standards and guidelines for physicians to review and analyze hospital care on a regular basis.[1,2]

In the 1950s, the American College of Surgeons joined within the American Hospital Association and American Medical Association to form the Joint Commission on Accreditation of Hospitals (JCAH). This group established minimum standards of performance for health care institutions. In the 1960s, to insure that care was reasonable and necessary, legislation was developed which required hospitals to set up utilization review procedures. By the early 1970s, Professionals Standards Review Organizations (PSROs) were developed by Congress to review medical practices and replace utilization review as a means of identifying appropriateness of services seeking reimbursement. PSROs were made up of local practitioners who determined the appropriate level of care for each patient through chart audit, length of stay and admission criteria. At the same time, private insurance also adopted criteria for appropriateness of care. In the late 1970s, JCAH and PSROs required that medical care evaluation studies be done by hospitals seeking accreditation and reimbursement.[3]

In the early 1980s, Peer Review Organizations (PROs) were established for physicians, and utilization review committees continued to function in health care facilities, each insuring appropriateness of services while attempting to contain costs. At this time, JCAH was renamed the Joint Commission on Accreditation of Health Organizations (JCAHO) and in turn has placed greater emphasis on quality assurance. Its focus is multidisciplinary, with standards of care established for all services. All disciplines in the health care organization are mandated to keep track of services in order to determine if they are being performed in an effective manner. In 1992 the term quality assurance was modified to include quality assessment and improvement standards. The revisions place greater emphasis on the role of hospital leaders in assessing and improving patient care, development of appropriate indicators of care and further clarifies the interdisciplinary nature of the monitoring process.[4,5]

In addition to those standards established by JCAHO, there are other methods available to determine quality. Industrial models utilize methods which focus on productivity, and profitability. Program evaluation, criteria mapping, periodic medical review and profile analysis are among those which have evolved in response to government regulations and accreditation requirements.[6] Most recently a management strategy known as total quality management (TQM) has been implemented in health care settings. This methodology is associated with improved product and service quality, improved productivity and morale and increased profitability. Health care organizations have begun to explore TQM incorporating quality improvement (QI) techniques with health care quality assurance and management.[7,8]

As a practical measure, it is reasonable to utilize the QA program established by JCAHO.[5] This program which is correctly referred to as quality improvement (QI), is applicable to a variety of health care settings and has a clearly defined procedure for implementation. Critical to this program is the establishment of an institutional QA plan. This plan mandates that the same level of care is provided throughout the institution. In turn, each area, service or department must develop an individual QA plan which is in keeping with the overall plan. It includes program organization, objectives, scope and mechanisms for overseeing the effectiveness of monitoring activities.

Monitoring Patient Care

There are ten steps which are necessary for effective monitoring and evaluation of the care provided. They are useful to follow when developing a QA program.

The first step is to assign responsibility for the monitoring and evaluation. Responsibility is assigned to a specific individual with authority to determine and implement QA activities and analyze compliance and follow-up. It is common that the director of occupational therapy (OT) has overall responsibility for an individual area. In turn, the director includes as many staff as possible in the process. Assisting in the process provides a greater understanding of the findings. Therapists providing direct treatment can delineate the scope of practice and identify important aspects of care. Assisting with data collection and analysis provides a greater understanding of the findings. Staff who assume ownership are better able to integrate these solutions into day-to-day practice.

The second step is to delineate the scope of care. All primary functions of the OT service should be identified, i.e., types of patients served, patient care delivered, e.g., diagnostic, therapeutic and preventive services, age groups of patients, basic clinical activities of practitioners and a definition of who provides care/services. For example, the hand management service provides care for adult patients with hand injuries in an ambulatory clinic, Monday through Friday, 8:00 a.m. to 5:00 p.m. The staff is comprised of hand surgeons and occupational therapists.

Step 3 identifies the important aspects of care provided, i.e., care which occurs frequently, is high risk or problem-prone. For example, in an acute care OT Department services which have high volume would be services which affect large numbers of patients, e.g., safety assessment and functional training for elderly patients living alone. An example of a high risk service is splinting, i.e., the patient is at risk for developing skin irritation or pressure areas. Problem-prone care are those aspects of care which can already be identified as frequently problematic, e.g., lack of compliance with the treatment regime such as missing scheduled treatment sessions.

In step 4, indicators of quality are developed. Indicators are defined, measurable dimensions of a specific aspect of care identified in Step 3. Indicators emphasize the appropriateness of care and outcome. This may include the adequacy, timeliness and effectiveness of an aspect of care. Examples of indicators are seen in Table 9-1.

In step 5, criteria or thresholds are set to determine how each indicator will be measured, i.e., what percentages or number of instances are acceptable to indicate quality care. The threshold set to measure the safety assessment indicator in Table 9-1 is set at 85%. In other words the expectation is that a safety evaluation is performed on 85% of all the elderly patients referred to OT who will return home alone.

The next step is to collect and organize data for each indicator. Using example 1 cited in Table 9-1, the patient medical record would be utilized for data collection. The medical record is a useful tool when monitoring indicators of care such as accurate and thorough documentation of functional training.

	Table 9-1 Indicators of Quality		
Important Aspects	**Indicators**	**Threshold**	**Methodology**
1. Safety assessment, functional training & documentation	Appropriate, timely & accurate safety assessment, functional training & documentation as evidenced by: 1. Safety assessment 2. Documentation of functional training and discharge planning.	85%	1. Quarterly random chart review of 20 records by OT. 2. Reports to OT Director, QM committee, hospital administration.
2. Hand Management referral	Appropriate, timely and accurate referral to Hand Management as evidenced by: 1. MD order signed, dated on all post surgical hand patients. 2. Post-op splinting on day of referral. 3. Follow-up treatment within 1 week of receipt of referral.	95%	1. Quarterly chart reviewed by Hand Management Service. 2. Reports as stated above.

Typically, there are four steps to the process:

1. Establish the standards of care to be provided.
2. Charts are reviewed to determine if practice meets the standards.
3. Charts that do not meet the standards are analyzed to identify issues and remedial action is taken and feedback given.
4. Follow-up is done if indicated by the findings.

Once data is organized, indicators which reach or exceed the pre-established threshold are evaluated to determine the area of concern (step 7). A new, more specific monitor may be developed to assess the problem. For example, the acceptable threshold for the indicator, Hand Management referral (Table 9-1, example 2) is 5%. The incidence of no referral for a given quarter is found to be 10%. Two new indicators are developed to determine the cause. One indicator monitors the lack of referral due to change in clinic medical staff in the summer (new fellows and residents); the second indicator monitors those due to lack of available appointments in Hand Management. At the end of the next quarter, data reveals that there is a long waiting time for follow-up appointments which results in patients not appearing for the appointment.

When the problem has been evaluated, action must be taken to resolve the problem (step 8). To continue the example of Hand Management referral, a task force is established

---

Table 9-2
Guidelines For Documentation of Quality Management Activities

---

Indicator:	Identify the aspect of care and clinical indicator being discussed.
Evaluation:	Identify the threshold, standard of acceptable care and actual performance. Outline what has been gleaned from the investigation of the issue.
Recommendations:	Describe what is being recommended to address the areas of concern identified through the review. If no recommendations are made, this should be stated.
Actions:	Describe the steps to be taken to ensure that recommendations are followed. Assign responsibility to a specific person or task force. If no action is necessary, this should be stated.
Follow-up:	Document plans to ensure that recommendations are followed and that these actions effectively address the issues identified. State the time frame for follow-up.

---

to examine the wait time for follow-up appointments and make recommendations to resolve the situation. Additional appointment times are established as recommended. Other action strategies may change behavior or identify the need for additional knowledge.

In step 9, the effectiveness of the action taken is assessed and the findings are documented. When the indicator Hand Management referral is monitored for the next quarter, and the threshold of 5% is not exceeded, it is determined that the task force has resolved the problem.

The last step, communication of relevant information, is the responsibility of the OT director. Typically, QM reports are sent regularly to the administrator of the organization and the QM Department and appropriate committees. Table 9-2 provides a suggested outline for how the report may be written. The QM Department may choose to make recommendations to other departments or key people as indicated by the findings presented. Most importantly, findings and follow-up must be shared with staff members. This can be done through staff meetings, individual meetings with staff involved with the project and written communication summarizing the findings with recommendations for future QM activities. Table 9-3 presents a schematic diagram of this 10 step monitoring and evaluation process.

Measures of quality must emphasize processes, not individuals. In this definition, process refers to a sequence of activities that transform inputs into final products, or outputs.[8] Process measures which focus on compliance with procedures such as activities which go on between practitioners and patients do not necessarily reflect all aspects of Quality patient care.[9] In fact, the current changes in the JCAHO monitoring and evaluation standards emphasize the need to assess quality improvement in patient activities. For example, the process by which patients are discharged. This is a departure from a discipline specific,

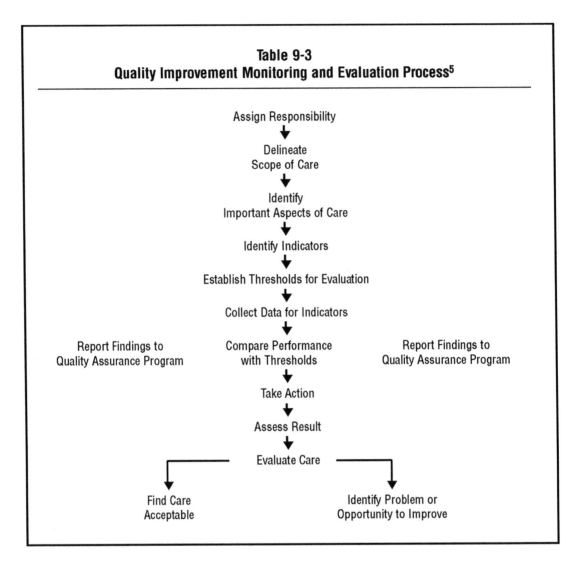

Table 9-3
Quality Improvement Monitoring and Evaluation Process[5]

problem oriented approach to one which emphasizes the integration of efforts to improve patient outcome. In this regard, effort must be directed at:

1. Leadership's role. Institutional leadership must take the lead in quality improvement.
2. Time and resources must be substantively invested in the quality care effort.
3. Respect for the health care worker must be reestablished.
4. An open dialogue between customers (patients) and suppliers (health care providers) must be maintained. The focus of quality improvement is on the customer.
5. Objective and theoretically grounded tools for improving processes must be utilized.
6. The institution must be organized for quality, using new managerial techniques which refocus the role of regulators to one of partners with caregivers in developing measurement tools used to evaluate quality improvement. Health care professionals, including physicians, must take an active role in specifying preferred methods of care.

7. Developing clear, scientifically grounded, continuously reviewed statements of process (how one intends to behave) are critical to quality improvement.

8. The key is to implement continuous quality improvement, with hospital-wide involvement, as well as participation of the physician's office practice.[3,5,10]

The success of quality management is based on how well quality care activities are conducted. Simply complying with regulations is not enough. Quality care findings must be meaningful to each practitioner. Current quality care practice is by no means the final step in the continually changing process to adequately define and measure quality care. Awareness of the legal and ethical issues which impact current health care practice is critical. Future quality management must ensure that quality results are a balance of these concerns as well as that of fiscal accountability.

References

1. Meisenheimer CG. *Quality Assurance: A Complete Guide to Effective Programs.* Rockville, MD: Aspen Systems, 1985.
2. Merry MD. What is quality care? A model for measuring health care excellence. *QRB.* 1987; 9:298-301.
3. Liang MH, Fortin P. Quality assurance and audit: lessons from North America. *Ann Rheum Diseases.* 1991; 50:522-525.
4. *Accreditation Manual for Hospitals.* Chicago: The Joint Commission on Accreditation of Healthcare Organizations, 1992.
5. *Quality Improvement for Hospital Clinical and Support Services.* Chicago: The Joint Commission on Accreditation of Healthcare Organizations, 1991.
6. Williamson JW. Future policy directions for quality assurance: lessons from the health accounting experiences. *Inquiry.* 1988; 25:67-77.
7. Kleefield S, Churchill WW, Laffel G. Quality improvement in hospital pharmacy department. *QRB.* 1991; 17(5):138-143.
8. Laffel G, Blumenthal D. The case of using industrial quality management science in health care organizations. *JAMA.* 1989; 262(20):2869-2873.
9. Donabedian A. The quality of care: how can it be assessed? *JAMA.* 1988; 260:1743-1748.
10. Berwick DM. Sounding Board: Continuous improvement as an ideal in health care. *N Engl J Med.* 1989; 320(1):53-56.

Questions/Case Studies

1. What are the most important services (key functions or aspects of care) that OT department provides? For whom are these services provided? What measures do you use to assess the performance of the important services?

Important Services (Aspects of Care)	Recipient(s) of Service	Measures (Indicators)
1.		
2.		
3.		
4.		
5.		

Questions/Case Studies (continued)

2. What threshold will be set for each measure (indicator)? Is this indicator so important that a threshold be set for 100% or 0%? What data source will you use for each indicator? Who collects the data? For this exercise, assuming that the threshold has been exceeded, what is the action plan to address the problem or opportunity for improvement? What follow-up is recommended for this action?

Measure (Indicator)	Threshold	Data Source	Who Collects	Action Taken	Follow-up
1.					
2.					
3.					
4.					
5.					

CHAPTER 10

Developing a New Occupational Therapy Program

Mary Jane Youngstrom, MS, OTR/L

Introduction

When faced with the task of conceptualizing, developing and proposing a new program for an occupational therapy department, the manager's initial response may be one of confusion and indecision. Where do you start? How do you think of feasible ideas for programs? What information do you need to support the establishment of a new program? How do you convince administration of the importance of the program and gain support for its implementation?

These are all important questions, and ones that need to be addressed within the program development process. Taken as a whole they may appear overwhelming, but approached in a step by step manner each question becomes an important stage in the overall process of program development.

The What, Why, and Who of Program Development

What is a program and what is program development? A program is a specifically designed service that is aimed toward a specific goal and is designed to achieve clearly defined outcomes or results. An occupational therapy department may have numerous programs within the department itself such as the stroke program, the developmental assessment program, or the community re-entry program. The department may be the only provider of service in a program or it may be a participant in a program which includes service providers from several disciplines. Program development is a step by step process that focuses on the planning and development of an idea that will lead to a new service in an OT department. It may be as limited as developing a new service in an already established department, such as starting a group feeding training program in a hospital's rehab unit. Or, it may be as comprehensive as designing a program of occupational therapy services in a newly opening psychiatric hospital.

Why are programs needed? Programs are needed to clearly focus effort and activity and to directly meet the needs of identified groups. When activities are organized into programs they often become more visible to other groups and help to increase understanding and utilization of occupational therapy services. For example, in one occupational therapy department, arthritis patients were referred for treatment on an inpatient basis but were rarely referred as outpatients. The department organized an outpatient arthritis program, clearly outlining treatment services and outcomes patients could expect. When physicians understood this program outpatient referrals increased.

Occupational therapists in management and staff positions are frequently faced with the need to develop new programs. The impetus for a new program may come from others, such as when the hospital board of directors decides to open an outpatient arthritis center and the OT manager is asked to develop the occupational therapy program for the center. Often the need for a new program will be recognized by an individual therapist, based on his or her day to day experiences with patients. An example would be when a therapist recognizes that his/her patients are not improving in their feeding skills as anticipated and decides to develop a special group mealtime program.

The rapidly changing health care environment may also encourage the development of new programs. Developing technology and advances in treatment techniques may prompt new programs. Within the past twenty years, significant advances in hand surgery techniques have fostered the development of specialized post-surgery hand therapy programs. Changes in patient populations admitted to an institution and identification of new diseases such as AIDS have prompted therapists to devise programs to meet the needs of these populations.

Lastly, sometimes new programs are developed to bring together services for clients in a new or more refined way that is more readily understood and accessed by the community. For example, an occupational therapy department may have provided preschool screenings on a sporadic basis, but after developing a specific preschool screening program was able to target more schools and provide an increased number of screenings as well as follow up consultation.

Who does the planning? The planning may be carried out by one person or a group of people. It is often helpful to involve several people or even a committee in the planning process in order to solicit a broad range of ideas and gain differing perspectives. In an occupational therapy department the manager or director often carries the official responsibility for program development. However, the responsibility for program development belongs to each therapist who identifies a need for change or sees an opportunity for improving care for his or her patients. Official responsibility for the development of a specific program may be delegated to a supervisor, senior therapist, or assigned to a committee. However, including others at some point in the development process is advisable in order to increase others' awareness of occupational therapy's role and acceptance of the proposed program changes.

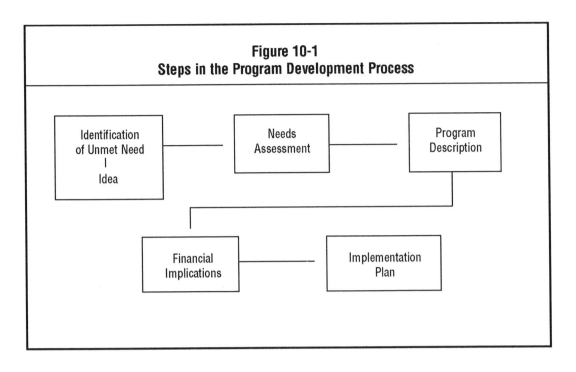

Figure 10-1
Steps in the Program Development Process

Overview of Steps

What does the occupational therapist do when faced with the prospect or need for starting a new program? Although initially it may appear to be an insurmountable task, the development of a program is a step by step process not unlike the treatment planning process—and therefore one familiar to occupational therapists.

When does program planning and development occur? It can occur at any time—more specifically when a need for a program change is noted. In some organizations planning cycles are formalized so that the opportunity for submission of new program ideas occurs at a routine time. This time is most often connected with the budget cycle. In other organizations a program proposal may be submitted at any time.

The program development process begins with an idea and ends with the implementation of the proposed program. In between these two points the planners engage in an objective and thorough analysis of the actual need for and justification of the program. The specifics of the program are outlined and described, and the costs and benefits of the program are identified. The steps of the process can be conceptualized as pictured in Figure 10-1. A description of each step follows.

Step 1—The Idea

Ideas for new programs generally spring from the recognition of an unmet need. The therapist who scans her environment and listens to and observes what is happening around her will discover many sources for ideas.

Patients and their families often know better than anyone else what their unmet needs are and are an excellent source of ideas. By watching patient responses and listening carefully to their concerns the therapist can often identify the underlying needs being expressed. The therapist who repeatedly listens to the spouses of her stroke outpatients express worry and concern about the ability of the husband or wife returning to driving would be using this approach. After listening to their concerns the therapist might identify a need for improved information about driving ability to be made available to patient and family. The therapist might propose that a specialized driving assessment program be developed to address this need.

Feedback from other health care providers can also prompt new ideas for programs. The nurses who repeatedly report to the occupational therapy department that patients are not following through with independent feeding skills after the initial occupational therapy training may prompt the department to consider a noon time group feeding program.

The community and its members are another source of ideas for new programs. Reading the newspaper and talking to individuals outside of the health care environment can broaden one's perspective and stimulate creative thinking. Involvement in school, church and community groups can open doors to ideas as well as collaboration. For example, repeated informal contacts with pre-school teachers in the community may reveal a need for formal developmental testing—a service an occupational therapist could provide.

Critically observing what is currently being done in a department or within one's practice can also give one clues as to unmet needs and present ideas for new programs. Analyzing information routinely collected in your department such as attendance/discharge records and continuous quality improvement reports can lead to ideas for new programs. For example, a quality improvement monitor which looks at amount of improvement in basic self care skills and which documents a low rate of improvement in dressing skills may prompt a department to start a special bedside dressing program. Likewise, analysis of outpatient attendance records which shows poor and irregular attendance by COPD patients may prompt a department to establish a more structured 8 week program using a group format to improve attendance and participation.

Ideas may spontaneously arise from various everyday contacts as described above or ideas for a new program may be more formally sought through a structured process using a marketing planning approach. This approach is outlined in Chapter 3 of this book on marketing and includes both an internal assessment (self audit to determine the department's strengths and weaknesses) and an external assessment (analysis of the consumer, other service providers and the overall environment). Many health care organizations now employ marketing specialists who can act as a resource to the occupational therapist. These specialists can assist in market analysis and identification of potential new programs. Other structured methods such as surveys sent to patients, family, and/or health care team members soliciting feedback and ideas on new programs or interviews with key referral sources and clients can be a springboard for new ideas.

During this step it is important to identify the unmet need as clearly as possible. Clearly but briefly describe:

- the target population
- the problem or unmet need
- the proposed program

As the idea begins to form the program planners also need to ask themselves what is the program's overall goal? What is the general thrust of the program? Defining a goal, even at this early stage will help to focus the purpose and direction of the program and will guide later steps in the process. For example, an occupational therapy department may decide to develop a work hardening program. Is the goal of the program to offer expanded services to current outpatients who are not returning to work quickly or is the goal to offer a service not readily accessible in the community to a broader population? Depending on the goal chosen, the target population and program scope and design may be very different. The goal selected at this stage is only tentative and may be modified and changed as more information is gathered.

The proposed program and its goal must be compatible with the organization's overall direction. Therefore, it is important to compare the proposed program goal with the organization's mission statement. A program that is not compatible with the organization's purpose will never be fully accepted or successfully supported in the sponsoring organization. As an example, an occupational therapy department in an acute care hospital decides that a stress management/wellness outpatient program is needed in their community. The mission of the hospital has been defined as providing state of the art medical care to acutely and chronically ill community members. The OT department is able to gather community support and even demonstrate through a survey a strong interest among community members. However, a comparison of the hospital's mission statement with the program's goal shows that the two are not compatible. The hospital's mission is to serve the acutely and chronically ill. The OT department's proposed program is directed toward serving the well community.

Clear definition of the target population, the problem, the broad program solution, and its initial goal prepare the way for Step 2.

Step 2—The Needs Assessment

The purpose of this step is to factually substantiate the need or problem you have identified in Step 1. The following three questions need to be answered:

1. What is the event of the given problem? How many individuals does it affect? How frequently does it occur? Is it expected to increase?
2. How and to what degree is this problem being addressed currently within the department or by others?
3. What are the factors that contribute to or sustain the problem?

The difference between the answers to questions 1 and 2 is the unmet need and will define the extent and size of the problem. The answer to question 3 will support whether your program idea directly addresses one or more of the factors contributing to the problem.

The planners begin by collecting data that specifies the size and scope of the problem. Sources of data might include departmental records, medical charts, and/or results of surveys and quality assurance studies. Interviews with individuals in the targeted population to be served or with primary referral sources who would use the new program can contribute to defining the extent and nature of the problem. Demographic information such as age, rate of occurrence of health problems and health status indicators is often available from health care regulatory agencies. Such data can be used to document the extent of the problem or of the targeted population. In the proposed driving assessment program example referred to earlier, the planners would want to identify how many patients treated in the last year would have been potential candidates. A survey of physicians requesting estimates of the number of patients they see per year who might be referred to the programs could also be taken. Both numbers would give planners an idea of exactly how many people might use the proposed program.

The existence of the problem needs to be supported by objective evidence such as statistics and figures which substantiate the level and frequency of occurrence. However, planners should not neglect to use statements of support from prospective clients or program users as well as other organizations or community groups who would agree with the need for the program.

It is important that the needs assessment take place as a separate step in the planning process. Having to substantiate a fledgling program idea with hard data will either convince or dissuade the planners of the need for the program. Without this step, which often acts as a "reality check," planners may proceed with more detailed program development and finally program implementation only to find that the program fails because the need was not as large as was anticipated. The process of gathering real facts about the extent of the problem can also lead the planners to modification of the original program idea which more directly addresses the actual need and will end up being more successful.

When the needs assessment is completed all the information and data should be analyzed. An accurate picture of the existing situation should emerge. The planners at this point determine if the facts support the need and if the need is large enough to justify spending additional time and resources on further program development planning. Assuming that the answer is yes, the planners proceed to Step 3.

Step 3—The Program Description

During this step of program development the program is outlined and described. The planners must take their idea and describe how the program will work and who will be involved. The overall scope of the program must be defined. The following six topics should be addressed.

Figure 10-2
Examples of Program Goals and Objectives

Program: **Community Re-entry Skills Program**

    Goal: To expand services to head injury in and outpatients by including community re-entry skill activities in their treatment regimen.

    Objective: 75% of the patients treated in the community re-entry skills program will demonstrate improved ability to handle themselves in a community setting.

Program: **Pediatric Mental Health Occupational Therapy Evaluation**

    Goal: To provide developmental screening for children hospitalized on the mental health unit.

    Objective: 85% of the patients referred to the pediatric mental health unit will receive developmental screenings.

Program: **Injured Worker Program**

    Goal: To increase occupational therapy's referral sources.

    Objective: Increase the number of contracts within area for the injured worker program by two within the next year.

---

1. **Goals and objectives.** The goal initially selected in step one should be re-evaluated in light of all the data collected in the needs assessment step. Does the data collected in the needs assessment support this goal? Or does the general goal and direction of the program need to be modified?

Once the goal is re-defined program objectives must be formulated. A goal statement for the program, which describes the general thrust of the program, has already been formulated. Now objectives, which are more specific and detail the results and outcomes to be achieved need to be identified. Objectives: a) should be relevant and related to the problem/need identified, b) should be stated in terms of results or outcomes of the program, c) should be measurable, and d) should be achievable. Some examples of goals and objectives for several different programs are described in Figure 10-2.

2. **Target population.** The specific population who will be served by the program should be described. Who exactly is the program to serve? Who should *not* be served? Factors to consider might include age, diagnosis, ability level, and location.

3. **Setting.** Where will the program take place? Will it take place in the hospital or the community? Is the space already allocated or will additional space need to be found? Briefly describe the basic physical requirements of the space needed, i.e., a large open room, three small office spaces, etc.

4. **Outline of program activities**. A detailed description of the activities and/or methods that will be used to achieve the objectives should be developed. What services will the O.T. department provide? Does the program include consultation, evaluation and/or treatment? Will educational activities with family and/or other team members be included in the program? The development of a flow chart detailing how the services will be organized and outlining how a patient will "flow" through the program can be a helpful tool in this process.

5. **Volume**. Based upon the extent of need ascertained during the needs assessment the demand for service to be provided by the program must now be projected. Volume or service demand frequently varies from month to month. Projections may be made on a monthly basis and plotted out for the first year of program operation. Typically volume for a new program will start out low and gradually increase as the program becomes established and recognized. In predicting volume it is important to be positive yet realistic. Volume projections can end up influencing the program's financial viability and acceptance.

6. **Resource utilization**. After the planners have outlined the activities and estimated the volume of work expected they are in a position to outline the resources the program will require. Resources include space, equipment, supplies, and staff.

Space—The proposed program may be housed in existing space, renovated space, or new space. The approximate square footage required and the general type of space needed should be delineated.

Equipment—Equipment is categorized into two types: capital equipment and non-capital or minor equipment. Capital equipment is generally considered to be any large item costing $500 or more which will last two or more years. Items such as desks, file cabinets, treatment tables, and some test kits are capital items. Smaller equipment items such as hand tools and adaptive equipment are non-capital items. Equipment needs will vary depending on the type of program and the volume anticipated.

Supplies—Supplies include all expendable items such as office supplies, test forms, splinting materials and media supplies. Supply needs will also vary depending on the type of program and volume anticipated.

Staff—Two decisions need to be made about staffing resources required—the kind of staff (OTRs, COTAs, aides, secretaries, etc.) and the number of staff. The kind of staff required will be determined by the services the program will offer and the skill level needed to perform the services. The number of staff needed can be determined by plotting out the hours needed to carry out patient treatment activities, documentation, meetings, and preparation/follow-up. It may be helpful to lay out a mock work schedule based on projected volumes. Time should be allowed for lunch and break times also.

Step 4—Financial Implications

The financial implications of a program include both the program's costs and revenues. At this point in the program development process the program is clearly outlined and it is time to allocate costs to the resources which will be used and to estimate what probable revenues or income may be.

Costs

Costs basically fall into two categories: 1) initial start-up costs, and 2) operating expenses. Start-up costs would include all supplies and equipment (both capital and non-capital) which will need to be purchased and available for use when the program begins. Renovation costs to the space to be used should be considered. If it will be necessary to hire staff or use current staff time to prepare for the program before it opens, these manhours and their costs should also be included as well as any training costs. Marketing and promotions costs also need to be included. Operating expenses are those costs accrued by the program after it begins. Ongoing supply, equipment, and staffing costs are included. Generally, operating expenses are estimated for the first year of operation.

Revenue

At this stage the planners must determine whether the program will be a revenue producing service or whether its costs will be absorbed by the department or organization. Some programs which may not involve direct patient treatment or for which reimbursement is not available may not be revenue producing. If the program will produce revenue, then fees for services provided must be established.

Different fees may be established for different services such as individual treatment, group treatment, evaluations, splints, etc., or fees already established by the department may be used. The AOTA Uniform Terminology document may be a helpful resource to guide decisions about categories of services to charge. If new fees are to be established the following information should be considered:

1. actual costs involved in providing the service
2. what reimbursers currently pay for services and policies regarding payment
3. what other providers charge for similar services

Consultation with the financial manager of the institution is recommended to determine whether fees charged should cover all expenses, a portion of expenses, or all expenses plus provide a profit. In most cases the fee needs to be high enough to cover costs and allow for a margin of profit, yet low enough to be within the range of charges allowed by reimbursers and/or charged by other providers in the area.

After the fees are established the total revenue is estimated by multiplying the volume estimated for each service times the fee charged for each service. Adding together the revenue produced for each service will provide the planners with the total revenue projected for the new program.

Comparison of Costs and Revenues

A direct comparison of cost and revenue will reveal that the program a) makes money, b) loses money, or c) breaks even (revenues cover costs). Depending upon the philosophy of the organization in which the program resides one or several of the above may be preferable. Program planners would be wise to be aware that this "bottom line" figure will often have a strong influence on the program's viability and acceptance within the organization. If the bottom line demonstrates a loss the program may need to be reconsidered by re-evaluating volume projections, costs, and fees for service.

Step 5—Implementation Plan

The last step of the program development process is the design of a plan for implementing the program. All facets of the program have now been described. The planners know where the program will take place, what supplies and equipment are needed and what staffing is required. They have wrestled with how the program will look and what different activities will occur within the program. Now the planners must sort out the separate tasks that must be accomplished to bring the program into being. As the tasks are identified they should be plotted along a time line with target dates for completion noted.

In the implementation plan, consideration should be given to the tasks that need to be carried out in the following areas:

Space preparation—The physical space where the program will be housed may need to be acquired, renovated or arranged. If the program is to be housed in current space some equipment may need to be moved and/or other changes made. Plans and target dates for moving will need to be made.

Supplies and equipment—Necessary items will need to be ordered in time to allow for delivery, installation and stocking before the start of the new program.

Activity preparation—The policies, procedures, and protocols for the activities which will be part of the program need to be developed. Although these may change after the program is underway the staff involved in the program need to think out some basic procedures ahead of time in order to direct their actions in the beginning of the program.

Staff preparation—Personnel to staff the new program will need to be recruited and hired. Job descriptions also need to be developed. Current and newly hired staff may need additional training if new skills are needed for the proposed program. Orientation to program goals, objectives, and protocols for all staff will be required before the program opens.

Promotion—Plans for marketing the program to clients and referral sources are essential for the success of the program. How are people to be notified about this new service? Is a brochure needed? Newspaper coverage? Individual contact with referral sources? The chapter on marketing in this book further discusses this topic.

Evaluation—A plan for evaluating the effectiveness and success of the program should be formulated as part of the implementation plan. Criteria for determining the success of the program and a procedure for collecting the necessary data need to be built into the plan. Two kinds of criteria should be considered—process evaluation criteria and outcome evaluation criteria. Process evaluation criteria will focus on the way the program has been conducted. For example, all evaluations were completed within two treatment sessions. Outcome evaluation criteria will focus on the results of the program. They measure the program's outcomes. For example, 75% of patients treated in the work hardening program will return to gainful employment by the completion of the program. The program's objectives, if they have been specifically and measurably written, should form the basis of the program's outcome evaluation.

Figure 10-3
Outline for a Written Program Proposal

I. Purpose and Justification
   A. Purpose of program
   B. Problem the program addresses
   C. Assessment of need

II. Description
   A. Program description
   B. Implementation plan

III. Analysis of Costs and Benefits
   A. Financial Implications
   B. Program Benefits
   C. Risks and uncertainties

IV. Summary and Conclusions

Writing the Program Proposal

Producing a written document that presents and summarizes all the thinking and planning of the program developers is the culmination of the process. The hard work is done. The planners now take their information and organize it for others to review. The written program proposal provides a record of the planning process and should answer all basic questions about the program's purpose, content and benefits. A suggested program proposal outline is presented in Figure 10-3.

Most of the information to be included in the written proposal has already been generated during the program development process. However, program benefits and risks and uncertainties have not been specifically addressed.

As the planners near the end of the program development process they should have a clear idea of the program's benefits and potential risks. The financial benefits have been clearly outlined under financial implications. They can be briefly summarized and restated here along with other quantitative benefits such as productivity, change in market share, or effectiveness. Qualitative benefits which may be more difficult to quantify should not be overlooked. The effect of the new program on the organization's image, influence, and quality of care may be significant. Risks and uncertainties associated with rapidly changing conditions or current problems might influence the viability of the program and should be noted. Changing government or reimburser policies, pending legislation, risk associated with being able to recruit staff are possible examples.

The Planning Process

Since the program development process is a sequential one and new information is being gathered and developed along the way there are several points at which the planner may pause to re-evaluate whether the program is still worthwhile and whether to continue the process. For example, if the needs assessment demonstrates that the actual need for or utilization of the proposed program would be minimal the planners may decide that further development of the program is unnecessary. Likewise, if during the program description step it becomes apparent that costs to set up the program are becoming excessive the planners may choose to stop the process or scale down their original idea to make it less costly.

The steps in the process have been presented in a logical sequence. However, in actuality steps may overlap or information acquired in one step may require the planners to go back to a previous step. Planning is a continuous process and is never truly completed in the sense that new information may require the planners to revise previous plans.

Conclusion

The program development process allows the planners to think through their ideas in a logical and comprehensive manner. Facts are gathered to support ideas and conclusions. The process allows the planners to anticipate problems and minimize failure. A program which has been well planned has a greater chance of running smoothly and being successful. Good planning is the cornerstone to effective programming.

Questions

1. A program is:
   a. Any activity carried out in an occupational therapy department
   b. An activity that involves patient treatment only
   c. A specially designed service aimed toward a specific goal
   d. All of the above

2. Ideas for new programs come from:
   a. The marketing department
   b. Patients and families
   c. Other health care providers
   d. All of the above

3. Which of the following statements does not describe the program development process?
   a. The process is composed of sequential steps
   b. Once started all the steps of the process must be completed
   c. The process allows the planners to anticipate possible problems
   d. The process requires the planners to support their ideas with factual data

4. Program development is the responsibility of:
   a. The department manager
   b. The senior supervising therapist
   c. The staff therapist
   d. All of the above

5. The step of the program development process in which the planners gather factual information to document the existence of the problem is called:
   a. The idea stage
   b. The needs assessment
   c. The program description stage
   d. The financial implications step

6. When the planner is describing the program in step 3, which of the following is not addressed?
   a. The program's benefits
   b. The outline of the program's activities
   c. The target population
   d. The program's usage of resources

7. The purpose of the needs assessment step is:
   a. To convince others of the need for your program
   b. To assess the needs of the patients targeted for your program
   c. To begin to market your program
   d. To factually support the extent of the problem your program will address

8. Which of the following factors should be considered when establishing fees?
   a. Costs involved in providing the service
   b. What others charge for the same or similar service
   c. What reimbursers will pay for the service
   d. All of the above

9. Which of the following is true about program goals and objectives?
   a. Goals and objectives are the same thing
   b. They should be consistent with the organization's direction and mission
   c. Once set they should not be changed
   d. They are nice to have but are not an important aspect of the program development process

10. The statement, "85% of the patients referred to the pediatric mental health unit will receive developmental screenings," is an example of which type of evaluation criteria?
    a. Process evaluation criteria
    b. Outcome evaluation criteria

Answers
1. c
2. d
3. b
4. d
5. b
6. a
7. d
8. d
9. b
10. a

Case Study 1

Shelley is an occupational therapist who works in a pediatric outpatient clinic treating children ages 4-14 with sensory integration dysfunction and mild to moderate developmental delays resulting in learning disabilities. Every summer for the last several years she has listened to the parents of her clients complain about the lack of available structured summer activities for their children. She has also noticed that the social skills and judgment of her clients are deficient and has struggled with how she could more effectively address these needs in her 1:1 therapy program. She decides that perhaps both of these needs could be addressed in a new program—a summer play camp offered in her outpatient clinic. Her target population would be children 6-11 years of age with developmental delays.

Shelley shares her idea with the occupational therapy manager who agrees that it has merit and asks her to develop a program proposal for the idea. As she begins thinking about her idea she defines an initial goal for the proposed program. It is: To study the need for a structured group program which would improve social skills in the developmentally delayed and learning disabled child.

To verify whether or need a need exists for her program Shelley conducts a survey of the parents whose children she has treated within the last three years. Survey response is overwhelmingly positive. Parents would be very interested in a summer program. She also contacts several local schools for the learning disabled and interviews their directors. The directors also confirm the need for such a program and are able to give her estimates of the number of children who might be appropriate and interested.

Based on the information gathered, Shelley confirms the need for the program and now begins to work out the details of the program's description. She refines her goal to: Provide a structured group experience for learning disabled children aimed at improving social skills. The specific objective of the program will be: To improve social skills as measured on a social skills indicator in 75% of the children participating in the program. She decides that her target population should include any learning disabled child in the community age 6-11. She proposes that the program be conducted in the gymnasium and recreation space of a nearby church. With equipment available from the clinic and the church further major equipment will not be needed, but some expendable supplies such as media supplies and cooking supplies will be needed. Shelley draws up a sample program of activities for the summer camp and decides she will propose running one 4 week session. After consideration of the kind of activities that will be conducted and the number of possible campers she decides that the program can be run with one OTR and an aide. Based on the information she received from her parent survey and interviews with school directors she estimates that 10-15 campers may be interested.

She now sits down with the department's manager and specifically outlines start-up costs and operating expenses. A fee for the camp session that will cover expenses plus make a small profit is set.

Together Shelley and the manager map out the implementation plan and develop a time line for sequence in which tasks to get the program running need to be accomplished.

The information that has been developed is compiled into a written proposal and submitted for approval.

Case Study 2

Ann is the manager of the occupational therapy department in a 400 bed hospital in a medium sized midwestern city. The hospital's board of trustees, responding to decreasing demands for inpatient services, has decided to expand the mission of the hospital to include outreach to nearby communities.

The hospital's occupational therapy department has had a tradition of attracting and retaining a capable and stable work force due to the variety of its programming and effectiveness of its management. However, fluctuating inpatient caseloads have lowered productivity.

As manager, Ann is aware of several smaller hospitals within a 70 mile radius that have been unable to recruit and retain OT staff. She sees an opportunity to support the mission of the hospital, make more efficient use of her staff's time, and assist hospitals in need of occupational therapy services. She proposes the development of a new program to provide contract occupational therapy services to area hospitals.

After discussing the proposed idea with her administrator, she proceeds to conduct a needs assessment by collecting data from area hospitals. She discovers three hospitals that have been unable to provide occupational therapy services for 5 of the last 9 months. The administrators estimate that their average caseload varies from 2-5 patients per day in each hospital. The administrators contacted appear interested in exploring a way to provide more consistent service.

Ann proceeds to outline the program description as follows:

Goal statement: To improve the availability of occupational therapy services in local medical institutions by providing outreach occupational therapy contract services.

Objective: Increase department revenues by 15% and staff productivity by 20%.

Target population: Patients referred to OT in area hospitals.

Setting: OT clinics in area hospitals.

Program Activities: Patient evaluation and treatment.

Volume: Approximately 6-15 patients will be treated per day at three different sites. Amount of therapist time required to carry out this activity is estimated at 6-20 hours per day plus travel time.

Resource Utilization: Space, equipment and supplies will all be provided by the host hospitals. One to one and one-half OTRs will be required to carry out the program.

Financial implications were next determined by comparing costs and projected revenues. Initial start-up costs were minimal, involving basically the time required to negotiate contracts with the three hospitals. Operating costs included the therapists' salaries, benefits and travel costs to the three facilities. Revenues were projected based on an hourly fee established for contract services. Multiplying the hourly fee times the estimated number of therapist hours required yielded the total revenue the program would generate. Revenues exceeded costs and therefore the program was considered to be financially viable.

A brief implementation plan was outlined which focused on orienting and preparing staff for contract work and outlining policies and protocols.

References

1. American Occupational Therapy Association. *Uniform Terminology for Occupational Therapy—Second Edition*. American Journal of Occupational Therapy. 12:808-815, 1989.
2. Anthony RN, Herzlinger RE. *Programming: New Programs, in Management Control in Nonprofit Organizations*. Homewood, Ill: Richard D. Irwin, Inc., 1975.
3. Budgen CM. Modeling: A Method for Program Development. *Journal of Nursing Administration.* 17:19-25, 1987.
4. Dignan MB, Carr PA. *Program Planning for Health Education and Health Promotion*. Philadelphia: Lea & Febiger, 1987.
5. Haw M, Claus E, Durbin-Lafferty E, Iverson S. Improving Nursing Morale in a Climate of Cost Containment. Part 2: Program Planning. *Journal of Nursing Administration.* 11:10-15, 1984.
6. Kiritz NJ, Mundel J. *Program Planning & Proposal Writing Introductory Version*. Grantsmanship Center. Los Angeles, CA (article reprint).
7. Mayer R. *Policy and Program Planning: A Developmental Perspective.* Englewood Cliffs, New Jersey: Prentice Hall, Inc., 1985.
8. McDonald P. *Program Development: Program and Project Planning and Review.* Boise, Idaho: Health Policy Analysis and Accountability Network, Inc., 1977.
9. Persly N, Slavin W, Albuny S. Marketing Rehabilitation Programs in Marketing Everybody's Business Symposium Digest. American Marketing Association, 1988, pp. 115-117.
10. Scammahorn G. Program Planning in Bair J, Gray M (eds.). *The Occupational Therapy Manager.* Rockville, MD: The American Occupational Therapy Association, 1985.
11. Twain D. *Creating Change in Social Settings: Planned Program Development.* New York, NY, Praeger Publisher, 1983.
12. Van de Ven A. Problem Solving, Planning and Innovation. Part I. Test of the Program Planning Model. *Human Relations.* 33:711-740, 1980.
13. Van de Ven A. Problem Solving, Planning, and Innovation. Part II. Speculations for Theory and Practice. *Human Relations.* 33:757-779, 1980.

Index